AI in Orthopedic Trauma Care 2

AI in Orthopedic Trauma Care 2

Advances in Intelligent Imaging, Decision Support, and Rehabilitation

Edited by

Abhishek Kumar
Priya Batta

iSTE

WILEY

First published 2026 in Great Britain and the United States by ISTE Ltd and John Wiley & Sons, Inc.

ISTE Ltd
27-37 St George's Road
London SW19 4EU
UK

www.iste.co.uk

John Wiley & Sons, Inc.
111 River Street
Hoboken, NJ 07030
USA

www.wiley.com

Library of Congress Control Number: 2026937210

British Library Cataloguing-in-Publication Data
A CIP record for this book is available from the British Library
ISBN 978-1-83669-138-9

The manufacturer's authorized representative according to the EU General Product Safety Regulation is Wiley-VCH GmbH, Boschstr. 12, 69469 Weinheim, Germany, e-mail: Product_Safety@wiley.com.

Contents

Preface

Artificial intelligence (AI) is transforming healthcare by enabling advanced data analysis, improved diagnostics and efficient clinical decision-making. In orthopedic trauma care, timely and accurate assessment of fractures and musculoskeletal injuries is critical for effective treatment and recovery. Recent developments in machine learning (ML), deep learning (DL) and medical imaging analysis are supporting clinicians in detecting injuries, planning surgeries and monitoring patient outcomes with greater precision.

AI in Orthopedic Trauma Care 2 presents recent research and practical applications of AI technologies in trauma management. This book brings together contributions from researchers and healthcare professionals to highlight innovative approaches that enhance patient care, efficiency and future developments in intelligent orthopedic systems.

May 2026

Preface written by Abhishek KUMAR and Priya BATTA.

Introduction

Orthopedic trauma care deals with complex injuries involving bones, joints and surrounding tissues that require rapid diagnosis and precise treatment planning. With increasing trauma cases worldwide, healthcare systems are exploring innovative technologies to improve clinical efficiency and patient outcomes. Artificial Intelligence (AI) has emerged as a powerful tool capable of analyzing medical images, patient records and large healthcare datasets to support clinical decisions. AI-based models can assist in fracture detection, injury classification, surgical planning and rehabilitation monitoring.

The integration of AI into orthopedic trauma care also promotes a more data-driven and personalized approach to treatment. By utilizing predictive analytics and intelligent algorithms, healthcare professionals can assess risk factors, anticipate complications and design patient-specific treatment strategies. AI-supported tools can enhance clinical workflows, reduce diagnostic errors and support surgeons in making informed decisions during complex trauma cases. As research and technology continue to evolve, collaboration between orthopedic specialists, data scientists and healthcare institutions will be essential to fully realize the potential of AI-driven solutions in improving trauma care, rehabilitation outcomes and overall quality of patient management.

Introduction written by Abhishek KUMAR and Priya BATTA.

This book explores the role of AI in transforming orthopedic trauma care by presenting research advancements, clinical applications and future directions for integrating intelligent systems into trauma management and patient-centered healthcare delivery.

1

Prediction of Fracture Union in Long Bones Using AI Models

The predictive capability for estimating healing time in long-bone fractures is vital for improving patient outcomes and preventing of complications in orthopedics. Delays or non-union fractures if left untreated may result in sustained disability, increased medical expenses and dysfunction. The current prediction techniques are primarily based on clinical examination, X-ray interpretation and bone-turnover blood tests, which are subjective and often inaccurate. Artificial intelligence (AI) and machine learning (ML) are promising solutions to current developments. The AI models include supervised learning algorithms, neural networks and ensemble approaches that analyze multi-dimensional and complex data that comprise patient demographics, fracture characteristics, surgical history, imaging and lab findings. The AI-based models are superior in prediction compared to traditional methods because they are able to identify subtle trends among these variables. This review sums up the recent findings on AI application to the healing of long bone fractures, such as important algorithms, data sources and clinical variables to be included in the model construction. It additionally provides discussion of how the imaging modalities (plain radiographs, CT, MRI) can be integrated with AI to increase the accuracy of the diagnosis, it also mentions such challenges as the quality of data, the explainability of models and their implementation in clinical practice. Lastly, the review shows that future AI-based decision support systems can personalize treatment, enhance clinical decision-making, and eventually improve the healing process.

1.1. Introduction

Long bone fractures, including those of the femur, tibia, humerus and forearm bones, are a significant clinical problem due to their frequency, severe complications and healthcare resource requirements (Jha et al. 2025). These injuries are caused by high energy impact such as car collisions or

---

Chapter written by Santosh TAKALE and Dalavi Surekha GORAKH.

height falls and low energy impact among the elderly who have weak bones. Early fracture healing is an essential step towards restoring functional status, preventing complications and reducing the social costs of prolonged rehabilitation.

The process of healing fractures is dynamic, involving inflammation, formation of a callus, ossification and remodeling. Success is determined by a vast number of factors related to patients including age, sex, comorbidities (e.g. diabetes or osteoporosis) and other lifestyle habits (e.g. smoking and nutrition) (Donié et al. 2024). The location, pattern, severity of fractures and nature of treatment (surgery or conservative care) are also factors that have a significant positive effect on outcomes. Delayed or non-union results in chronic pain, chronic immobility, loss of functional ability and possibly another surgery.

Conventional fracture healing monitoring incorporates clinical evaluation, image and laboratory findings. Skilled clinicians frequently consider pain relief, limb function restoration and weight-bearing capacity as signs of healing, however, these are subjective and cannot be related to the underlying biology (Razavi et al. 2025). Serial X-rays are by far the most commonly used method to evaluate callus formation and cortical continuity, but they are subject to interpretation bias, and the initial indicators of healing are delicate. Advanced imaging modalities, such as CT and MRI, provide greater detail, particularly in complicated or joint fractures but are not routinely used because of cost, radiation exposure, and limited availability.

Predictors of healing have also been examined through measuring blood levels of bone turnover markers, such as serum alkaline phosphatase, osteocalcin and C-terminal telopeptide (Morgan et al. 2024). Even though these biomarkers are objective, they have a low rate of clinical utility because they vary among individuals and there are no standardized cut-offs. Due to this fact, the traditional methods are often inadequate for early and precise prediction of fracture union, particularly in high-risk or complex cases.

ML and AI have become potentially valuable technologies that can eliminate these constraints (Jha et al. 2025). AI systems have the ability to break down multi-dimensional data that incorporates patient demographics, fracture features, radiographies, surgical and laboratory findings to come up with predictive models of union. Supervised learning algorithms including random forests and support vector machines are also capable of determining important predictors of delayed or non-union, whereas deep learning models, especially convolutional neural network models, are able to automatically learn features based on imaging data, thereby enhancing the prediction of delayed or non-union.

The current literature proves that AI-based models have been capable of delivering personalized prognoses, aiding clinical decision-making and streamlining patient care (Misir 2025). Using the combination of sources of data, AI algorithms can prioritize patients based on their level of risk, foster early interventions and even decrease the risk of repeated imaging. Although effectively showing good results, issues of data heterogeneity, small sample sizes, model explainability and its use in standard clinical practice continue to hamper large-scale adoption.

The main purpose of this chapter is to extensively review AI applications in predicting fracture union in long bones. It covers the nature of AI models used, predictive variables and data sources, integration of imaging modalities with AI analysis, predicted model performance and lack of guidance on the main challenges and the future of AI implementation in clinical use. It is hoped that this review will provide orthopedists, researchers and AI developers with a clear vision of the advantages and limitations of AI-based fracture union prediction and contribute to positive patient outcomes and tailored fracture treatment.

1.2. Types of AI models for fracture union prediction

Models of fracture union prediction are becoming increasingly dependent on AI. They are able to analyze intricate data and identify patterns that can easily escape clinicians.

There are four broad categories of AI models, which comprise supervised and deep, unsupervised, and hybrid or ensemble models (Elkohail et al. 2025). All types have strengths which are dependent on data and clinical circumstance.

The most common supervised learning models in the case of fracture union prediction are supervised learning models. They are trained using known datasets in which outcome; union or non-union, is known. Random forest, support vector machine, gradient boosting and logistic regression are some of the models that have been effective in predicting healing. As an example, the random forest manages various data and identifies the most significant predictors of fracture such as the type of fracture, patient age and method of fixation to provide clear outcomes that can be useful in clinical decision-making (Cha et al. 2023).

DL is proficient in picture-based prediction. Convolutional neural networks are able to automatically extract high-level features of radiographs, CT or MRIs and reveal signs of subtle healing without any labeling. Recurrent neural networks and long short memory units are better adapted to time-series data, for example, time-varying imaging trends or time-varying lab trends, allowing time-dependent healing modeling (Lin et al. 2023).

Unsupervised learning is less common but can identify hidden patterns without labeled data. Methods such as k-means clustering, hierarchical clustering and principal component analysis cluster patients together based on fracture characteristics, healing capacity or risk factors. These can guide the development of future models and improve understanding of patient heterogeneity (Liu et al. 2023).

Hybrid and ensemble approaches combine multiple models to enhance accuracy and robustness. For example, combining random forest with gradient boosting or integrating ML with deep networks can enhance performance and generalizability. These approaches help mitigate overfitting, which is particularly helpful for achieving reliable predictions in clinical practice (Yüce et al. 2025).

Compared to conventional tools, AI models have added benefits: they can handle multidimensional datasets of size, model nonlinear interactions between variables and give quantitative results. Still, some problems exist, including the need for extensive and high-quality data, overfitting and transparency of some DL models which complicates interpretability, exist (Karthik et al. 2025). In spite of these concerns, AI predictions have performed better than the traditional tests, which opens up the possibilities of a revolution in treating long bone fractures.

1.3. Data sources and predictive variables

The quality of the data and its diversity is crucial to the correctness of AI predictions. The demographics of the patient such as age, sex, BMI and comorbid conditions such as diabetes, osteoporosis, as well as smoking, dependably correlate with the healing results (Schulz et al. 2025). The age factor and some health conditions postpone bone regeneration; this is why such variables are necessary in predictive modeling.

The nature of the fracture greatly impacts union. Biological healing depends on variables, which include location, type (transverse, oblique, comminuted), degree of displacement and involvement of soft tissues (Takahashi et al. 2023). High energy or complex fractures are risk factors which predispose patients to delayed or non-union. Risk is stratified using AI models to inform treatment decisions.

Surgical specifics are the most essential factors of healing. Such variables as the fixation technique (intramedullary nailing, plating, external fixation) and the quality of reduction, as well as perioperative care, influence the outcome (Engels et al. 2024). This data can be incorporated into AI to assess the effect of surgical decisions on union and provide information upon which to determine the postoperative care or prompt intervention in the case of high-risk patients.

Visual images are a source of valuable information to AI prediction. X-rays, CTs and MRIs detect the fracture structure, callus, bridging of the cortical bone and bone density (Namireddy et al. 2024). Radiomics uses quantitative image features to create patterns that clinicians otherwise would have overlooked, thus increasing accuracy and objectivity.

Biochemical bone turnover markers, such as alkaline phosphatase, osteocalcin and C -terminal telopeptide, give insight into the bone physiology (Liu et al. 2024). Individual variability is also present, but integrating such markers with demographic, clinical and imaging data enhances AI performance, particularly for patients with complex comorbidities or bone metabolic imbalances.

1.4. Integration of imaging with AI

The key aspect of fracture assessment is medical imaging, and the combination of the latter with AI has led to a significant enhancement of fracture union predictions. The traditional methods of radiographs are the most accessible and least expensive forms of healing follow-up. Serial X-ray AI models may be used to identify otherwise hard-to-see evidence of callus formation and cortical bridging, which may be missed by a human viewer and thereby identify even delayed union early (Chen et al. 2025b).

Computed tomography (CT) provides three-dimensional images of a high-resolution view of the bone structure, fracture fragments and even the process of healing in detail. With the aid of AI algorithms, it is possible to analyze volumetric and textural features based on CT information, and such measures have been called the callus volume, bone mineral density and cortical continuity. Such objective measurements enhance the accuracy of fracture-healing measurements compared to traditional interpretation by itself (Chen et al. 2025a).

Magnetic resonance images (MRIs) are better in the assessment of soft-tissue involvement, bone-marrow edema and vascularization on the fracture site. DL algorithms will analyze MRI images to evaluate the bone and tissue in the area, and the results allow us to have a holistic understanding of factors aiming at affecting union (Capkin et al. 2025). AI can serve more comprehensive healing outcome prediction, especially when applied in conjunction with MRI data and clinical and demographic data, especially in cases of complex or high-risk fractures.

Radiomics: the methodical mining of quantitative imaging features – also known as Radiomics – is an effective method of combining AI with imaging data. Radiomic features present texture, shape, intensity and Einstein at the fracture site which is all associated with biological healing potential. Radiomics increases sensitivity and specificity of models when it is fed in together with ML algorithms, allowing early and precise predictability of union or non-union (Fang et al. 2025).

Altogether, AI-based imaging modality integration shifts the approach to both assessing and predicting subjects to a more sustainable, data-driven perspective. Radiographs, CT and MRI as a part of AI, are used to complement each other, and they are incorporated into AI-based prognoses to provide robust and individualized outcomes. Radiomics and DL technologies, specifically, will revolutionize the management of fractures because it will be possible to provide an accurate, timely and personalized approach to fracture management.

Table 1.1 presents AI models, data sources and predictive performances in long bone fracture union.

AI model category	Representative algorithms	Primary Data inputs	imaging integration	Predicted outcomes	Reported performance trends
Supervised machine learning	Random forest, SVM, gradient boosting, logistic regression	Demographics, comorbidities, fracture type, fixation method	Optional (radiographic features)	Union versus delayed/ non-union	Accuracy often >85%; good interpretability
Deep learning (image-based)	CNNs	Serial X-rays, CT, MRI	core input modality	Early union prediction, callus formation	High AUC (≈0.90+), reduced observer bias
Temporal models	RNNs, LSTM	Longitudinal imaging and lab data	Serial imaging	Healing progression over time	Improved dynamic prediction
Unsupervised learning	k-means, PCA, hierarchical clustering	Multidimensional clinical data	Not mandatory	Patient subgroup identification	Risk stratification support
Hybrid / ensemble models	RF + GBM, ML + DL combinations	Clinical + imaging + lab data	Strong integration	Robust union prediction	Reduced overfitting, higher generalizability
Radiomics-based AI	ML + radiomic features	Quantitative CT/MRI/X-ray features	Essential	Biological healing potential	Higher sensitivity and specificity

Table 1.1. *AI models, data sources and predictive performance in long bone fracture union*

1.5. Performance of AI models in predicting fracture union

AI models predictive of fracture union have been assessed in a number of studies and have proven to be significantly accurate and applicable in the clinical setting. ML algorithms including random forests and gradient boosting machines have demonstrated high predictive accuracy (often over 85%) in identifying patients likely to achieve timely union versus those at risk of delayed or non-union (Leister et al. 2023). These frameworks combine the multidimensional clinical, demographic and fracture-specific variables and provide strong predictions that are effective over traditional statistical methods.

Image-based predictions of fracture healing are best done using DL (CNNs, in particular). Recently, CNNs, trained on serial radiographs, CT or MRI images, are able to detect the initial signs of callus formation and cortical bridging, with great sensitivity and specificity in predicting fracture union (Erne et al. 2025). Other studies have given an area under the curve measurement of more than 0.90, which means that the discriminating ability is high. Notably, DL models automatically manipulate multifaceted imaging aspects, which lowers the use of manual interpretation and minimizes interobserver diversity.

Comparative studies involving AI models and conventional clinical evaluation reflect the superiority of AI models in predictive accuracy. Traditional systems, such as radiographic scoring systems and clinical assessment, do not usually have predictive capacity regarding early onset and are subject to analyst bias (Donié et al. 2024). On the contrary, AI can give objective, quantitative predictions, which can be used to stratify risks and intervene in time. Indicatively, patients who are identified by AI as high-risk non-union can be monitored closer or provided with additional treatment options, which may lessen complications and enhance results.

There are a number of clinical trials that demonstrated in practice the use of AI models in fracture management. Tibial and femoral fractures have shown high accuracy with the use of predictive models that combine patient demographics, fracture features, operation procedures and radiographic outcomes to predict union (Potty et al. 2023). These works show that it is possible to integrate AI-based decision support into orthopedic practice and present valid data on personalized predictive approaches to optimize patient care.

Altogether, there is high potential with AI models to predict fracture union due to their high accuracy, sensitivity and objective assessment of intricate data. Although issue such as data heterogeneity and model interpretability still exist, the presented performance of ML and DL models seems to indicate that AI can play a major role in improving the management of fracture and enhancing the outcomes of patients.

1.6. Challenges and limitations

The models of AI offer high potential in predicting the formation of a fracture, yet there are various obstacles that prevent them from being implemented on a regular basis in clinical practice. The quality and heterogeneity of the data that they are trained on is a significant problem. Dependable performance is necessary: the large and heterogeneous, high-quality datasets, and most studies are based on the small and single-centered sources, which are unlikely to be generalized (Raj et al. 2024). The variation in imaging protocols, patient demographics and the method of collection of data further complicates it and can be a source of bias in any prediction.

The second barrier is the inability to be interpreted. DL models are often regarded as a black box, and it is difficult for clinicians to understand why a specific prediction was arrived at (Park et al. 2024). This lowers trust and decreases acceptance. Explainable-AI techniques are still becoming available; however, there are few standard methods to use in fracture-prediction models.

There are also practical issues associated with the implementation of AI into practice. The models should be compatible with the available hospital information systems, PACS and EHRs (Raj et al. 2024). It needs deployment, hardware, staff training and also a change in workflow, which may be challenging in resource-constrained environments. Real-time decision support should be usable and accurate enough to not clutter the clinicians.

There are ethical, legal and privacy problems complicating the issues. Through AI, very sensitive patient data are usually handled, and this can be problematic in terms of confidentiality, security and consent (Wang et al. 2025). Medical AI regulations are in their development stages, and it is not clear how wrong predictions are liable. Fair performance in different populations is needed in order to prevent bias to exacerbate care disparities.

To conclude, AI has a chance to be used in predicting fracture union; however, addressing these issues is critical to use this technology safely and ethically in the clinic. Enhanced data quality, the creation of models that can be analyzed and uninterrupted integration of workflows as well as clear regulatory and ethical standards are the major steps that will enhance broader adoption in orthopedics.

1.7. Future directions

Future success will rely on large and multi-centered datasets. Obtaining data from a large number of institutions enhances the size of the sample, its diversity and applicability in a variety of settings and patient demographics (Gupta et al. 2025). These datasets generate powerful algorithms that work in clinical practice and minimize bias in single-center studies and increase clinical relevance.

It is also important to have explainable AI. Interpretability of models enhances trust in the clinicians and simplifies daily use. Such techniques as attention maps, feature-importance lists and model-agnostic frameworks assist clinicians to visualize what variables or imaging characteristics make predictions (Gupta et al. 2025). XAI enhances the trust and advances the clinical education.

Fractures can be changed with the help of AI, combining them with telemedicine and IoT devices. With remote patient monitoring and an AI analysis of imaging and clinical reports, it is possible to predict delayed union in a timely manner, minimize unnecessary visits and perform prompt intervention (Lin et al. 2025). Longitudinal mobility, load-bearing and adherence data may be included in wearable sensors and provide insights useful to predictive modeling and provide real-time individualized evaluation of the healing process.

Individualized forecasting models will transform orthopedic care. The combination of demographic, clinical, imaging and biochemical data can generate personalized healing curves and risk factors based on the AI models. These predictions would be used to make more specific interventions – when to start the weight-bearing, what should be fixed or whether adjunctive therapy is necessary, which benefits the outcomes and saves resources (Lin et al. 2025). Further research, extensive validation including external datasets, and close collaboration between clinicians and data scientists will be essential to unlock the full potential of AI in fracture union prediction.

1.8. Conclusion

Having accurate predictive capability for long bone healing is essential in enhancing patient outcomes, informing treatment choices, and reducing costs associated with delayed or failed healing. Conventional approaches using clinical evaluation, plain radiography, imaging and biochemical indicators are insufficient. They are not objective and are likely to vary, and in most cases are not able to predict the healing at an earlier stage. This is changing with the introduction of AI, as numerous data types, including patient demographics, fracture characteristics, surgical information, imaging features and laboratory findings, are integrated into models that provide objective and personalized decisions. All forms of ML supervised, DL and ensemble have demonstrated good potential in terms of predicting fracture union with precision, sensitivity and specificity. Convolutional neural networks and other forms of DL are capable of analyzing imaging data automatically. They also detect fine patterns that human eyes might overlook showing the extent to which the healing is taking place. Prediction is further enhanced by additional radiographs, CT scan and MRI, as well as radiomic features to AI workflows. This assists in time-based intervention and individual therapy. Yet, challenges persist. There is great variability in data, small sample sizes may be used, models may be black box, it is difficult to connect new workflows to practice and ethical issues come up. All these barriers will be overcome by multi-center datasets, explainable AI models, telemedicine connections and customizable predictive models. The clinical adoption of AI tools requires these steps to be taken. Overall, the capacity of AI to predict fracture union provides a perspective of improvement in orthopedics. They can improve the results, streamline the process of making decisions and advance personalized medicine in terms of a fracture management tool.

1.9. References

Capkin, S., Kilic, A.I., Cici, H., Akdemir, M., Marasli, M.K. (2025). Machine learning models for predicting tibial intramedullary nail length. *BMC Musculoskeletal Disorders*, 26(1), 395.

Cha, Y., Kim, J.T., Kim, J.W., Seo, S.H., Lee, S.Y., Yoo, J.I. (2023). Effect of artificial intelligence or machine learning on prediction of hip fracture risk: Systematic review. *Journal of Bone Metabolism*, 30(3), 245.

Chen, T., Chen, J., Liu, H., Liu, Z., Yu, B., Wang, Y., Zhao, W., Peng, Y., Li, J., Yang, Y. et al. (2025a). Integration of longitudinal load-bearing tissue MRI radiomics and neural network to predict knee osteoarthritis incidence. *Journal of Orthopaedic Translation*, 51, 187–197.

Chen, Y., Liu, R., Zhang, C., Xue, B., Yuan, Y., Wang, C., Wang, R., Zu, W., Jiao, R., Fang, X. et al. (2025b). Virtual physical therapist system using full-chain patient data – Focusing on rehabilitation of orthopedic lower limb postoperative. Preprint. doi: 10.21203/rs.3.rs-5901666/v1.

Donié, C., Reumann, M.K., Hartung, T., Braun, B.J., Histing, T., Endo, S., Hirche, S. (2024). Predictive model development to identify failed healing in patients after non–union fracture surgery. In *46th Annual International Conference of the IEEE Engineering in Medicine and Biology Society (EMBC)*, 15 July, 1–4.

Elkohail, A., Soffar, A., Paul, A., Radu, L., Ahamed, M.W., Swealem, A., Sha, A.A., Veetil, H.H., Millat, M.S., Shah, R. (2025). Artificial intelligence in bone fracture detection: A review of evidence, limitations, and clinical integration. *Cureus*, 17(11), e97674. doi: 10.7759/cureus.97674.

Engels, S.M., Kamat, P., Pafilis, G.S., Li, Y., Agrawal, A., Haller, D.J., Phillip, J.M., Contreras, L.M. (2024). Particulate matter composition drives differential molecular and morphological responses in lung epithelial cells. *PNAS Nexus*, 3(1), pgad415.

Erne, F., Mühlberger, L., Ihle, C., Ehnert, S., Histing, T., Nüssler, A.K., Maurer, E. (2025). The impact of cardiovascular diseases on postoperative complications in orthopedic trauma patients. *Diagnostics*, 15(13), 1576.

Fang, L., Pan, Y., Zheng, H., Li, F., Zhang, W., Liu, J., Zhou, Q. (2025). A study on predicting the efficacy of posterior lumbar interbody fusion surgery using a deep learning radiomics model. *Academic Radiology*, 32(9), 5339–5352. doi: 10.1016/j.acra.2025.05.026.

Gupta, P., Shen, H.J., Patel, K., Guo, R., Heinz, E.R., Manyam, R. (2025). Artificial intelligence for predicting 30-day mortality after surgery for femoral shaft fractures: A retrospective study. *Indian Journal of Anaesthesia*, 69(6), 606–614.

Jha, G., Dhanjal, R., Malasani, S., Karunakaran, A.V., Malasani Sr, S., Karunakaran, A. (2025). Deep learning in scaphoid fracture detection and healing prediction: A systematic review of artificial intelligence applications in hand surgery. *Cureus*, 17(11), e97900. doi: 10.7759/cureus.97900.

Karthik, D., Betancourt, V.V., Madhukar, S., Huda, M., Cerdas, M.G., Sunil, A., Imam, B., Nasir, W., Ali, S., Qureshi, M. et al. (2025). Radiological innovations for monitoring bone regeneration and fracture healing. *Cureus*, 17(11), e97659.

Leister, I., Haider, T., Vogel, M., Vastmans, J., Langthaler, P., Mattiassich, G., Christ, A., Etschmaier, M., Eijkenboom, A., Burghuber, J. et al. (2023). A predictive model to identify treatment-related risk factors for odontoid fracture nonunion using machine learning. *Spine*, 48(3), 164–171.

Lin, C., Liang, Z., Liu, J., Sun, W. (2023). A machine learning-based prediction model pre-operatively for functional recovery after 1-year of hip fracture surgery in older people. *Frontiers in Surgery*, 10, 1160085.

Lin, Y., Xu, Y., Zhou, S., Liu, J., Zhang, M., Zhang, B., Chen, H. (2025). Updated advances on drugs and bone-targeting nanoparticles for osteoporosis therapy: Carrier materials, modification, function mechanism, and applications – A systematic review. *Pharmaceuticals*, 18(12), 1809.

Liu, X., Miramini, S., Patel, M., Ebeling, P., Liao, J., Zhang, L. (2023). Development of numerical model-based machine learning algorithms for different healing stages of distal radius fracture healing. *Computer Methods and Programs in Biomedicine*, 233, 107464.

Liu, L., Cai, B., Liu, L., Zhuang, X., Zhao, Z., Huang, X., Zhang, J. (2024). Research on the morphological structure of partial fracture healing process in diabetic mice based on synchrotron radiation phase-contrast imaging computed tomography and deep learning. *Bone Reports*, 20, 101743.

Misir, A. (2025). Artificial intelligence in orthopedic trauma: A comprehensive review. *Injury*, 56(8), 112570.

Morgan, G.T., Low, L., Ramasamy, A., Masouros, S.D. (2024). A novel strain-based bone-fracture healing algorithm is able to predict a range of healing outcomes. *Frontiers in Bioengineering and Biotechnology*, 12, 1477405.

Namireddy, S.R., Gill, S.S., Peerbhai, A., Kamath, A.G., Ramsay, D.S., Ponniah, H.S., Salih, A., Jankovic, D., Kalasauskas, D., Neuhoff, J. et al. (2024). Artificial intelligence in risk prediction and diagnosis of vertebral fractures. *Scientific Reports*, 14(1), 30560.

Park, J.Y., Lee, S.H., Kim, Y.J., Kim, K.G., Lee, G.J. (2024). Machine learning model based on radiomics features for AO/OTA classification of pelvic fractures on pelvic radiographs. *Plos One*, 19(5), e0304350.

Potty, A.G., Potty, A.S., Maffulli, N., Blumenschein, L.A., Ganta, D., Mistovich, R.J., Fuentes, M., Denard, P.J., Sethi, P.M., Shah, A.A. et al. (2023). Approaching artificial intelligence in orthopaedics: Predictive analytics and machine learning to prognosticate arthroscopic rotator cuff surgical outcomes. *Journal of Clinical Medicine*, 12(6), 2369.

Raj, M., Ayub, A., Pal, A.K., Pradhan, J., Varish, N., Kumar, S., Varikasuvu, S.R. (2024). Diagnostic accuracy of artificial intelligence-based algorithms in automated detection of neck of femur fracture on a plain radiograph: A systematic review and meta-analysis. *Indian Journal of Orthopaedics*, 58(5), 457–469.

Razavi, A.H., Hemmati, M., Nafisi, N., Mirahmadi, A., Laiwala, S., Keko, M., Vaziri, A., Rodriguez, E.K., Nazarian, A. (2025). Mechanobiology-guided machine learning models for predicting long bone fracture healing across diverse scenarios. *Computers in Biology and Medicine*, 196, 110683.

Schulz, A.P., Kowald, B., Münch, M., Seide, K., Weinrich, N., Barth, T., Kienast, B. (2025). Long-term evaluation of bone healing monitoring using an instrumented plate with measurement sensors (smart implant) over 10 years. *Sensors*, 25(18), 5779.

Takahashi, S., Terai, H., Hoshino, M., Tsujio, T., Kato, M., Toyoda, H., Suzuki, A., Tamai, K., Yabu, A., Nakamura, H. (2023). Machine-learning-based approach for nonunion prediction following osteoporotic vertebral fractures. *European Spine Journal*, 32(11), 3788–3796.

Wang, J., Wang, Y., Ren, J., Li, Z., Guo, L., Lv, J. (2025). Emerging applications of feature selection in osteoporosis research: from biomarker discovery to clinical decision support. *Journal of Bone and Mineral Research*, 40(10), 1106–1113.

Yüce, A., Yaşar, H., Misir, A. (2025). Can fracture non-union be predicted using deep learning? *Exploration of Musculoskeletal Diseases*, 3, 100790.

2

Osteoporosis Risk Assessment in Fragility Fractures Supported by AI Analysis

Osteoporosis is a chronic bone disorder which weakens bones and increases exposure to fracture. Fragility fractures are the result low-energy impact (when the fall is from standing height) and usually involve the hip, spine, wrist and proximal humerus. These injuries result in high morbidity, mortality and healthcare expenses particularly for older adults. Despite available diagnostic methods and treatment, osteoporosis is poorly diagnosed or poorly managed following a fragility fracture. This results in a high risk of getting further fractures. Traditional risk assessment methods are widely used but have limitations in sensitivity, accessibility and individual accuracy, particularly in bone mineral density (BMD) testing and clinical prediction models. Artificial intelligence (AI) is a relatively new approach capable of enhancing osteoporosis risk prediction. The AI techniques examined include machine learning (ML), deep learning (DL) and the analysis of large, multi-dimensional datasets, including clinical history, imaging, biomechanical measurements and laboratory tests to determine fracture risk with greater precision. In addition to aiding opportunistic screening, automated fracture recognition and patient-specific risk stratification of already fractured patients, AI systems support clinical decision-making in this area. This chapter reviews risk assessment of osteoporosis in fragility fractures with emphasis on AI-driven methods. It discusses current diagnostics, AI image analysis, predictive modeling, decision-support system and implementation challenges. The implementation of AI in care pathways may improve early diagnosis, secondary fracture prevention and patient outcomes.

2.1. Introduction

Osteoporosis is a skeletal system disorder that is characterized by a decrease in bone mass, worsening microarchitecture and a decrease in bone strength. Such alterations cause risk of fracture an injury frequently affecting older generations in the global population, particularly postmenopausal

---

Chapter written by Sandip R. PATIL and Chavan Vikrant U.

women or old men (Meena and Sankar 2021). The global high prevalence of fractures has increased due to aging, and increased life expectancy, posing a major problem to the population in terms of cost and health. Osteoporotic fractures, also known as fragility fractures, are caused by low-energy impact, which would not break a normal bone (Kanis et al. 2020). The most common sites include the hip, spine and wrist, and proximal humerus that have a specific clinical outcome and functional repercussions.

Fragility fractures often lead to subsequent fractures. Hip fractures are associated with high morbidity and mortality. The one-year mortality rate in elderly patients with comorbidities is approximately 30%. Survivors may also become dependent requiring unending rehabilitation or care in institutions (Dyer et al. 2017). Vertebral fractures often go undiagnosed because they may be asymptomatic. However, they can later lead to persistent pain, spinal deformity, loss of height, impaired lung function, and reduced quality of life. (Dyer et al. 2017; Larsson 2021). Distal radium and proximal humerus fractures also make life more difficult and increase the chances of other accidental bone fractures. The fracture cascade is a strong predictor of subsequent fractures following an initial fragility fracture (Larsson 2021). The risk of a second fracture increases sharply within the first two years after the initial fracture, highlighting the need for rapid identification, assessment, and treatment of osteoporosis.

Although effective diagnostic and therapeutic interventions exist, osteoporosis remains underdiagnosed and undertreated particularly following a fragility fracture, a condition referred to as the treatment gap (Ali et al. 2024). Contributing factors include lack of access to BMD testing, inadequate care pathways, inconsistent post-fracture assessment guidelines and inadequate clinician and patient awareness (Ali et al. 2024). In most systems, chronic bone health is not given priority, which results in delayed or no osteoporosis diagnosis. Thus, patients are discharged without adequate risk stratification, measuring of BMD and commencing medication, which continues putting them at risk of fractures in the future.

The traditional methods of assessing osteoporosis risk use the bone mineral density (BMD) values derived from DXA and clinical tools such as FRAX and QFracture (Sato et al. 2022). DXA provides a quantitative analysis of BMD of the lumbar spine and proximal femur in the form of T-scores. Although BMD is useful in predicting fracture risks at the population level, it is not very sensitive in predicting risk at the individual level. A significant portion of individuals who experience fragility fractures do not fall below the osteoporosis threshold based on BMD alone, indicating the need for additional risk evaluation strategies. Clinical aids such as FRAX use age, sexuality, history of fractids, steroids, smoking, alcohol and other disorders to estimate the likelihood of fracture within 10 years. However, such models use standardized risk weights and population assumptions, therefore, failing to detect individual fracture risk, bone quality or fall risk (Sato et al. 2022).

Recent AI developments provide new opportunities for assessing and treating osteoporosis. Imaging, clinical, demographic, genetic and biomechanical datasets are analyzed using AI techniques, including ML, DL, and typically involve large and multi- or multi-dimensional datasets. AI is more accurate in predicting fracture risk than traditional risk prediction because it identifies complex patterns among the risk factors. Medical imaging AI has the opportunity to test bone health using regular radiography or CT scans, identifying undiagnosed osteoporosis in patients presenting with fracture (Langsetmo et al. 2023). AI systems can also enable individualized risk stratification, continuous monitoring and identification of patients at high risk of secondary fracture, allowing timely intervention and improved quality of care.

The use of AI in osteoporosis care pathways is of particular importance to patients with fragility fractures. These are high-risk individuals, and timely diagnosis and intervention can significantly reduce the likelihood of subsequent fractures and associated complications (Langsetmo et al. 2023). AI risk assessment can benefit an individual by automating and standardizing post-fracture assessment, enhancing diagnostic precision and providing clinicians with data-driven advice. In addition, AI can be used to assemble brittle liaison services and clinical psyche assistance to improve follow-up, use resources more effectively and decrease the workload of suppliers.

2.2. Fragility fractures and osteoporosis: clinical significance

The most clinically important indicator of the osteoporosis condition and the existence of bone weakness is fragility fractures. They are typically caused by little trauma and disproportionately occur in the aged, particularly, in post-menopausal women and old men (Tanaka 2021). The usual locations include hip, spine, distal radius and proximal humerus, and each location leads to varying degrees of functional deficiency and long-term disability.

The worst form of fragility fracture is hip fracture as it is fatal, resulting in loss of independence and excessive healthcare expenditure. The mortality rate on a hip fracture within one year is still highly alarming, and most of those who survive end up having permanent mobility loss that renders them dependent on institutional care (Guo et al. 2025). Vertebral fractures are usually missed as they are not always symptomatic but result in long-term pain, deformity of the spine, impaired lung functions and low quality of life (Adams et al. 2022). The probability of experiencing further vertebral fractures and non-spinal fractures is also increased by a vertebral fracture.

The risk of having a fracture is high following the experience of a fragility fracture – this is referred to as the fracture cascade. Research indicates that individuals that experience a single osteoporotic fracture face a high risk of experiencing additional fractures particularly during the first two years following the initial trauma (Li et al. 2021). A high-risk condition warns us of the need for quick and precise evaluation of osteoporosis following a fracture.

Although there is a clear correlation between the risk factors of fragility fracture and osteoporosis, most patients are not evaluated and treated according to the underlying condition. The gap in the post-fracture treatment process is a global issue which can be attributed to low levels of awareness, disjointed treatments and insufficient screening guidelines (Aibar-Almazán et al. 2022). In the majority of cases, orthopedic and trauma teams focus on acute fracture management with minimal inclusion of osteoporosis evaluation into routine practice.

Fracture liaison services were developed to eliminate this gap by offering systematic assessment and treatment following a fracture. They increase the treatment and diagnosis rates, but they are still unevenly implemented and are restricted by the quantity of resources (Åkesson et al. 2022). The implementation of AI-enhanced solutions can improve the quality of care for fragility fractures through patient identification, risk stratification, and timely referral to osteoporosis evaluation.

Clinical, imaging and demographic data when combined can assist AI systems in identifying osteoporosis at an early stage in patients with fragility fractures, as well as speed up the provision of timely interventions, reducing the likelihood of secondary fracture, and enhancing long-term outcomes (Li n.d.).

2.3. Conventional osteoporosis risk assessment methods

Traditional methods of assessing the risk of osteoporosis include a BMD test and a history of clinical risk factors. The standard test is the dual-energy X-ray absorptiometry (DXA) due to its use of a standardized procedure, low-radiation dose and high epidemiologic likelihood (Prince et al. 2020). DXA is able to measure BMD at critical locations – the lumbar spine and the proximal femur, which are closely correlated with fracture risk. T-score levels recommended by the WHO are used in diagnosis and treatment.

DXA, although popular, has significant limitations. BMD is just a component of bone strength that lacks information on bone quality, micro-architecture, geometry and material characteristics. As a result, a significant number of fragility fractures develop in individuals of osteopenic, even normal BMD (Kanis et al. 2023). This deficiency is notably among older persons, and that of secondary osteoporosis where the chances of fracture are also influenced by factors other than bone density.

Frax and QFracture clinical risk models are based on DXA and incorporate additional non-skeletal factors. These programs are an approximation of 10-year fracture risk based on age, sex, fracture history, steroid use, lifestyle and comorbidity of choice, and may include BMD where it exists (Kanis et al. 2023). They have better risk stratification at the populace level, yet adopt definite algorithms based on the epidemiologic cohort, which might fail to mention the specifics of a person.

Conventional assessment has barriers to access and use. The distribution of DXA machines is not even, and they are concentrated in regions with low and middle income, which causes delay or missed diagnosis (Reid and Billington 2022). DXA is not used extensively even in the wake of a fragility fracture since the care pathways are disjointed and there is a lack of co-ordination between orthopedics and bone-metabolism professionals.

Other instruments offer more information on the bone quality. The review provides valuable insights into the aspects of vertebral fracture, trabecular bone score and advanced imaging techniques. T trabecular bone score is a score based on DXA images as an indirect measure of trabecular micro-architecture and is useful in predicting fracture in combination with BMD (Kong et al. 2021). Its use is limited due to cost, software requirements, and the need for clinician expertise.

Fracture risk prediction can be supported by biochemical bone-turnover markers. Bone-turnover markers are limited by biological variability and have limited predictive value when used alone for fracture prediction (Vivas, n.d.). These limitations highlight the need for more holistic, dynamic, and personalized risk assessment, particularly in patients with fragility fractures, where timely identification of high-risk individuals is essential (Corrao et al., 2023). These findings are summarized in Table 2.1, which compares conventional and AI-based osteoporosis risk assessment methods.

Aspect	**Conventional risk assessment**	**AI-based risk assessment**
Primary tools	DXA-derived BMD, FRAX, QFracture	Machine learning, deep learning models
Data sources	BMD values, limited clinical risk factors	Multimodal data (clinical, imaging, demographics, laboratory data)
Bone quality assessment	Limited (primarily bone density)	Advanced assessment including bone microarchitecture, geometry, radiomics
Imaging utilization	Dedicated DXA scans	Opportunistic screening from X-ray and CT scans
Vertebral fracture detection	Often underdiagnosed, manual reporting	Automated detection using AI algorithms
Individualized risk prediction	Population-based estimates	Personalized and dynamic risk stratification
Sensitivity for fracture prediction	Moderate; many fractures occur outside osteoporosis BMD thresholds	Higher predictive accuracy demonstrated in multiple studies
Accessibility	Limited by DXA availability	Increased accessibility through routine imaging
Clinical workflow integration	Separate from acute fracture care	Integrated into fracture liaison services and CDSS
Secondary fracture prevention	Often delayed or missed	Early identification and automated alerts for intervention

Table 2.1. *Comparison of conventional and AI-based osteoporosis risk assessment methods*

2.4. AI in medical imaging for osteoporosis

Diagnosis and evaluation of fractures relies heavily on medical imaging, and the significance of image tests has increased significantly due to AI technology. Convolutional neural networks and deep learning are capable of processing involved imaging data with a high level of accuracy equivalent to or exceeding that of a human specialist (Rodrigues et al. 2021). This feature is notable in osteoporosis whereby subtle structural alterations may be overlooked in a regular review.

Opportunistic screening is the most significant use of AI. Computer tomography (CT) scans acquired to study other issue traumas, imaging of the abdomen or cancer staging carry with them a wealth of data on bone density and structure. The vertebral bodies can be automatically segmented, and volumetric BMD can be calculated without additional radiation or time by AI algorithms (Li et al. 2025). This permits clinicians to screen large groups of patients that would not otherwise obtain specialized BMD testing, particularly those with fragility fractures.

AI-based vertebral fracture identification will deal with a significant care gap. Vertebral fractures are underreported due to being asymptomatic or really because radiology processes lack time. The DL models, when trained on large datasets of images, are dependable in detecting and categorizing the presence of vertebral fractures in radiograph and CT images, minimizing bias in the decisions of the observers and increasing the rate of detection (Keshtkar et al. 2025). The clinical significance of early detection is due to the fact that the presence of vertebral fractures increases the likelihood of developing new fractures and death.

Another important development in AI is known as Radiomics. Radiomics finds numerous quantitative features in images that extrapolate bone texture, shape, as well as spatial heterogeneity. These characteristics depict trabecular and cortical micro-architecture of more than bare measures of density (Calicchio et al. 2025). Radiomic data can be fed into ML models to enhance the ability to predict fracture risks, as well as differentiate patients who do not have osteoporotic fractures.

AI analysis is also useful with magnetic resonance imaging (MRI) and high-resolution techniques. AI is able to analyze bone marrow structure, depending on the orientation of the trabecula, and their cortical thickness giving a complete picture of bone quality (Chang and Chung 2022). Despite being more frequent in the studies at present, these approaches exemplify the opportunities of non-ionizing imaging to contribute improved osteoporosis risk assessment.

2.5. ML models for fracture risk prediction

ML has become an important component of AI-based osteoporosis studies. It is a fracture risk predictor which uses high-dimensional complex data. Conventional statistical models rely on a few preoperative assumptions and linearization. Conversely, ML algorithms identify nonlinear relationships and weak patterns between several risk factors (Liu et al. 2023). This plays a pivotal role in osteoporosis where the risk of fractures is a product of interaction between skeletal, clinical, behavioral and environmental factors.

Fracture risk prediction by researchers is used with a wide variety of ML algorithms, including random forests, gradient boosting machines, support vector machines and artificial neural networks. These models use a combination of factors such as age, sex, comorbidities, medication use, falls, lab findings and radiographic imaging features (Avanzo et al. 2024). A growing body of studies, including systematic and non-systematic analyses, demonstrates that ML models outperform traditional tools such as FRAX in discrimination and calibration, especially in high-risk fragility fracture groups.

DL is an expansion of ML that autonomously acquires hierarchical manifestations of raw data. Invented to work with imaging and longitudinal clinical data, deep neural networks discover a latent pattern related to bone fragility and the probability of fractures in the future that traditional feature extraction can overlook (Kim et al. 2025). They are greatly potent in case they are trained using substantial electronic health record materials, and community groups allowing customized and dynamic risk identification.

Continuous updating of risks is one of the benefits of the ML-based fracture prediction. ML models improve risk estimates in real-time when new patient data is available, for example, follow-up imaging of new clinical status changes (Muse and Topol 2021). It is a dynamic style that is particularly effective when the risk is likely to change as quickly as health does in the post-fracture period.

Despite these good results, ML models have a weak interpretability and clinical trust performance. Most advanced models are so complicated that they form a black box, making it difficult for clinicians to understand how the prediction was formed. Explainable AI, based on algorithms such as feature-importance ranking, SHAP values and attention mechanisms, helps to address this issue (Kim et al. 2025). These methods demonstrate the influence of each risk factor and increase the confidence of the clinician that they have made an informed choice.

ML-based fracture prediction risk helps to provide at-risk, individualized care to osteoporosis patients. It helps to detect patients that may potentially be benefiting from early intervention although they may not be at the threshold of diagnostic standards. ML models can significantly enhance the prevention of secondary fractures and the more resource-effective distribution of efforts in terms of fragility fracture treatment by offering more precise, personalized risk stratification (Wang et al. 2023).

2.6. AI-supported clinical decision systems in fragility fractures

The clinical decision systems (CDSS) based on AI are used to convert the advanced risk models into practical clinical practice among fragility fracture patients. They integrate ML outputs with electronic health records, imaging platforms and clinical workflows such that clinicians get real-time decision support (Sato et al. 2022). The AI-based CDSS can be used to engage in osteoporosis management to recruit high-risk individuals and initiate timely treatment, supporting the appropriate diagnostics.

An important role of AI-enhanced CDSS is a reduction in the post-fracture treatment gap. One thing that happens with the treatment of patients with fragility fracture is that only the acute injury is addressed, and the osteoporosis underlying is often overlooked. At the time of admission or discharge, AI systems automatically screening the data of patients warn clinic staff about the need to measure osteoporosis or refer to a fracture liaison service (Kanis et al. 2020). This computerized detection enhances clinician awareness and supports consistent secondary fracture prevention strategies.

In fracture liaison services, AI-based CDSS enhance care coordination, by ranking patients according to their individual fracture risk. They use models that integrate clinical, imaging and demographic data, allowing service providers to optimally distribute resources and target individuals who are at the most risk of subsequent fractures (Vivas n.d.). Automated reminders and follow-up prompts also improve adherence to recommended evaluation and treatment plans.

CDSS facilitate individualized treatment planning caused by AI. The systems can assist clinicians in selecting appropriate pharmacologic and non-pharmacologic interventions by adding fracture risk predictions to patient-specific factors, including comorbidities, renal function, medication history and fall risk (Chang and Chung 2022). Dynamic risk review enables clinicians to provide real-time adjustment of treatment, which promotes the management of long-term osteoporosis.

Despite these advantages, challenges remain. The key to successful implementation of AI-assisted CDSS is seamless integration into existing clinical workflows without causing alert fatigue. The systems should be easy to use, clear, and aligned with clinicians' needs to ensure acceptance and adoption. Explainable AI methods are essential for creating trust by clarifying how recommendations are generated (Wang et al. 2023).

Avoiding stagnation in terms of AI models is also important since monitoring and updating AI models should be performed on a regular basis in response to changing clinical practices. Carefully constructed and introduced, AI-assisted CDSS have the potential to significantly improve the detection of osteoporosis, enhance secondary fracture prevention and improve outcomes for patients with fragility fractures.

2.7. Challenges, ethical considerations and data limitations

The potential of AI in enhancing the risk assessment of osteoporosis in patients with fragility fractures is high, though a number of challenges have to be overcome to achieve safe, effective, and equitable clinical implementation. The first among them is the requirement for high-quality and standardized data. Large quantities of well-annotated information is necessary to train AI algorithms and certify their predictions. Osteoporosis-related data are often distributed across imaging archives, electronic health records, and clinical registries, which can lead to gaps, inconsistencies, and bias (Liu et al., 2023). Variations in imaging protocols, diagnostic criteria, and clinical documentation further limit the generalizability of findings.

Another significant problem is population bias. Most AI models are trained using data covering a small geographical area or a single health system that is not reflective of patients. Ethnicity, socioeconomic status, co-morbidities and care access may influence the fracture risk and presentation of osteoporosis. In cases where such factors have not been included in training data, the models may result in biased predictions and increase health inequities (Avanzo et al. 2024). This means that external appraisal within different populations is a prerequisite to clinical implementation.

The clinical acceptance of model interpretability is also a hindrance. DL models can be highly precise, however they are typically black boxes, which means it is difficult to understand how a prediction was made. This form of secrecy hinders trust and adoption.

To address the issue of increased transparency enabling clinicians to learn the reasons behind every prediction, explainable-AI techniques, including feature attribution and visual explanation applications, have been created (Kim et al. 2025). The tradeoff between a model's complexity and interpretability is not fully resolved to date.

Ethics and laws are also main issues in the deployment of AI. Patient privacy, data security and informed consent are paramount when working with large datasets that are going to be combined. The governance systems should clearly define responsibility and accountability, especially where AI plays a role in determining diagnosis or treatment (Muse and Topol 2021). Regulation of AI-based medical devices is evolving, and extensive prospective validation is required to demonstrate safety, clinical utility and cost-effectiveness of these devices.

Implementation of AI within regular operations present's technical challenges. The tools should be integrated into the current health-information systems and designed to support clinicians rather than overwhelm them. Continuous performance monitoring and frequent model updates should be conducted because the clinical practices and patient population evolve

(Wang et al. 2023). These challenges can be resolved using multidisciplinary collaboration, adherence to ethical standards and rigorous validation, enabling AI to unlock its full potential in osteoporosis diagnosis fragility fracture management.

2.8. Conclusion

Osteoporosis has continued to be a major cause of fragility fractures, as well as increased morbidity, mortality and socioeconomic burden. Fragility fractures provide a prime opportunity to detect individuals who are vulnerable to future fractures, but osteoporosis is often underdiagnosed and undertreated in this context. The traditional risk assessment tools can be used although they are limited in sensitivity, accessibility, and personalization.

The introduction of AI in osteoporosis risk assessment represents a significant advancement in the management of patients with fragility fractures. AI-based imaging analysis can automatically identify fractures, opportunistically estimate BMD, and assess bone microarchitecture with unprecedented detail. Machine learning algorithms can integrate clinical, imaging, and demographic data to generate more accurate and individualized risk predictions.

AI-based decision support systems can also help bridge the post-fracture treatment gap through systematic identification, assessment, and management of osteoporosis within routine care pathways. Although these developments are promising, challenges such as data quality, model explainability, ethical considerations, and clinical integration must be carefully addressed.

To ensure effective implementation, standardized datasets, transparent and explainable algorithms, robust validation, and close collaboration between healthcare systems, clinicians, and data scientists are essential. As AI technologies continue to advance, their thoughtful and responsible application in osteoporosis care has the potential to transform fragility fracture management, enhance secondary fracture prevention, and ultimately improve patient outcomes.

2.9. References

Adams, J., Nowels, C., Corsi, K., Long, J., Steiner, J.F., Binswanger, I.A. (2022). HIV risk after release from prison: A qualitative study of former inmates. *Journal of Acquired Immune Deficiency Syndromes*, 57(5), 429–434.

Aibar-Almazán, A., Voltes-Martínez, A., Castellote-Caballero, Y., Afanador-Restrepo, D.F., Carcelén-Fraile, M.D., López-Ruiz, E. (2022). Current status of the diagnosis and management of osteoporosis. *International Journal of Molecular Sciences*, 23(16), 9465.

Åkesson, K.E., Ganda, K., Deignan, C., Oates, M.K., Volpert, A., Brooks, K., Lee, D., Dirschl, D.R., Singer, A.J. (2022). Post-fracture care programs for prevention of subsequent fragility fractures: A literature assessment of current trends. *Osteoporosis International*, 33(8), 1659–1676.

Ali, A., Huszti, E., Noordin, S., Ali, U., Sale, J.E. (2024). Examining treatment targets and equity in bone-active medication use within secondary fracture prevention: A systematic review and meta-analysis. *Osteoporosis International*, 35(9), 1497–1511.

Avanzo, M., Stancanello, J., Pirrone, G., Drigo, A., Retico, A. (2024). The evolution of artificial intelligence in medical imaging: From computer science to machine and deep learning. *Cancers*, 16(21), 3702.

Calicchio, F., Epstein, E., Boussoussou, M., Vattay, B., van Rosendael, A., Newlander, S., Kolossváry, M., Szilveszter, B., Maurovich-Horvat, P., Marques, H. et al. (2025). Impact of technical, patient-related and measurement variables on serial Hounsfield unit-based quantitative coronary plaque analysis in computed tomography: Time for a new chapter. *European Heart Journal-Imaging Methods and Practice*, 3(1), qyaf014.

Chang, E.Y. and Chung, C.B. (eds) (2022). Musculoskeletal imaging of the older population, an issue of radiologic clinics of North America. In *Musculoskeletal Imaging of the Older Population, An Issue of Radiologic Clinics of North America*. Elsevier, Amsterdam.

Corrao, G., Biffi, A., Porcu, G., Ronco, R., Adami, G., Alvaro, R., Bogini, R., Caputi, A.P., Cianferotti, L., Frediani, B. et al. (2023). Executive summary: Italian guidelines for diagnosis, risk stratification, and care continuity of fragility fractures 2021. *Frontiers in Endocrinology*, 14, 1137671.

Dyer, S.M., Crotty, M., Fairhall, N., Magaziner, J.S., Beaupre, L.A., Cameron, I., Sherrington, C. (2017). A critical review of the long-term disability outcomes following hip fracture. *Innovation in Aging*, 1(suppl_1), 736.

Guo, J., Shi, L., Shi, K., Dai, R., Wang, J., Li, Y. (2025). A nomogram for one-year risk of death after hip fracture. *Frontiers in Medicine*, 12, 1500049.

Kanis, J.A., Cooper, C., Rizzoli, R., Reginster, J.Y. (2020). Scientific Advisory Board of the European Society for Clinical and Economic Aspects of Osteoporosis (ESCEO) and the Committees of Scientific Advisors and National Societies of the International Osteoporosis Foundation (IOF). Correction to: European guidance for the diagnosis and management of osteoporosis in postmenopausal women. *Osteoporosis International*, 31(4), 801.

Kanis, J.A., Harvey, N.C., Liu, E., Vandenput, L., Lorentzon, M., McCloskey, E.V., Bouillon, R., Abrahamsen, B., Rejnmark, L., Johansson, H., Danish Primary Hyperparathyroidism Study Group (2023). Primary hyperparathyroidism and fracture probability. *Osteoporosis International*, 34(3), 489–499.

Keshtkar, A., Karimi, A., Atighi, F., Yazdanpanahi, P., Naseri, A., Khajepour, A., Salehi, M., Sarikhani, Y., Dabbaghmanesh, M.H. (2025). Artificial intelligence applications in osteoporosis: A comprehensive review of screening, diagnosis, and risk prediction. *Shiraz E-Medical Journal*, 26(12) e162399.

Kim, C., Gadgil, S.U. and Lee, S.I. (2026). Transparency of medical artificial intelligence systems. *Nature Reviews Bioengineering*, 4(1), 11–29.

Kong, S.H., Hong, N., Kim, J.W., Kim, D.Y., Kim, J.H. (2021). Application of the trabecular bone score in clinical practice. *Journal of Bone Metabolism*, 28(2), 101.

Langsetmo, L., Schousboe, J.T., Taylor, B.C., Cauley, J.A., Fink, H.A., Cawthon, P.M., Kado, D.M., Ensrud, K.E., Osteoporotic Fractures in Men (MrOS) Research Group (2023). Advantages and disadvantages of random forest models for prediction of hip fracture risk versus mortality risk in the oldest old. *Journal of Bone and Mineral Research Plus*, 7(8), e10757.

Larsson, B. (2021). Predictors of bone fragility in older women. Associations in older women between risk medications and measurements of physical function, bone microstructure and fracture risk. Thesis, Göteborg University.

Li, N. (2023). Osteoporosis, (bone) fractures and fracture liaison services: Health-related quality of life, clinical and economic outcomes. Doctoral Thesis, Maastricht University. doi: 10.26481/dis.20230912nl.

Li, N., Hiligsmann, M., Boonen, A., Van Oostwaard, M.M., De Bot, R.T., Wyers, C.E., Bours, S.P., van den Bergh, J.P. (2021). The impact of fracture liaison services on subsequent fractures and mortality: A systematic literature review and meta-analysis. *Osteoporosis International*, 32(8), 1517–1530.

Li, Y., Zhang, B., Lu, F., Zou, Z., Tian, Z., Zhang, X., & Zhang, J. (2025). Analysis of intrinsic contributing factors in geriatric tibial plateau fractures using extended finite element method. *Journal of Biomechanics*, 194, 113060. doi: 10.1016/j.jbiomech.2025.113060.

Liu, X., DuMontier, C., Hu, P., Liu, C., Yeung, W., Mao, Z., Ho, V., Thoral, P.J., Kuo, P.C., Hu, J. et al. (2023). Clinically interpretable machine learning models for early prediction of mortality in older patients with multiple organ dysfunction syndrome: An international multicenter retrospective study. *The Journals of Gerontology: Series A*, 78(4), 718–726.

Meena, K.V. and Sankar, A.R. (2021). Biomedical catheters with integrated miniature piezoresistive pressure sensors: A review. *IEEE Sensors Journal*, 21(9), 10241–10290.

Muse, E.D. and Topol, E.J. (2021). More than meets the eye: Using AI to identify reduced heart function by electrocardiograms. *Med*, 2(7), 791–793.

Prince, R., Khoo, B., Brown, K., Lewis, J. (2020). Differences in femoral neck and trochanteric structure in elderly women prior to hip fracture: Role in hip fracture prediction. *Journal of Bone and Mineral Research*, 38(6), 869–875.

Reid, I.R. and Billington, E.O. (2022). Drug therapy for osteoporosis in older adults. *The Lancet*, 399(10329), 1080–1092.

Rodrigues, J.A., Krois, J., Schwendicke, F. (2021). Demystifying artificial intelligence and deep learning in dentistry. *Brazilian Oral Research*, 35, e094.

Sato, Y., Yamamoto, N., Inagaki, N., Iesaki, Y., Asamoto, T., Suzuki, T., Takahara, S. (2022). Deep learning for bone mineral density and T-score prediction from chest X-rays: A multicenter study. *Biomedicines*, 10(9), 2323.

Tanaka, Y. (2021). Managing osteoporosis and joint damage in patients with rheumatoid arthritis: An overview. *Journal of Clinical Medicine*, 10(6), 1241.

Vivas, L.P. (n.d.). Escore de osso trabecular como método de avaliação da qualidade óssea em pacientes com síndrome de cushing. Master's Thesis, Federal University of Minas Gerais, Belo Horizonte.

Wang, X., Chan, Y.S., Wong, K., Yoshitake, R., Sadava, D., Synold, T.W., Frankel, P., Twardowski, P.W., Lau, C. et al. (2023). Mechanism-driven and clinically focused development of botanical foods as multitarget anticancer medicine: Collective perspectives and insights from preclinical studies, IND applications and early-phase clinical trials. *Cancers*, 15(3), 701.

3

Postoperative Alignment Assessment After Total Knee Arthroplasty with AI Assistance

Total knee arthroplasty (TKA) is considered one of the most effective orthopedic surgeries in the management of end-stage knee osteoarthritis. Proper alignment of the postoperative position is critical to the survival of implants, biomechanical performance and patient-reported functional performance. Conventional evaluation features manual radiographic measurement, which is affected by inter- and intra-observer errors, waste in the workflows and a poor predictive capacity. Innovations in artificial intelligence (AI), and in particular, machine learning and deep learning have provided automated, objective and repeatable assessment consents. This chapter aims to discuss the use of AI-based technologies in the assessment of TKA alignment. It is a summary of the research on AI models based on imaging, such as radiography and computed tomography, as well as three-dimensional imaging convolutional neural networks. The combination of AI and navigation systems, robots and clinical decision-support systems is addressed. The validation plans, clinical performance indicators and comparisons in assessing alternative use compared with traditional methods are investigated. The most important issues, including dataset bias, regulatory approval, interpretability and adoption barriers, are also discussed. A summary of the latest advances and perspectives indicates that the assessment based on AI will enhance the precision of the diagnosis, make the assessment more regular and provide more tailored approaches to rehabilitation, which is why the review seems to have a transformative effect on the overall performance of the TKA in the long term.

3.1. Introduction

Total knee arthroplasty (TKA) has emerged as one of the most fundamental surgical surgeries on degenerative knee osteoarthritis and rheumatoid arthritis, as well as other degenerative joint diseases. As the

Chapter written by Channapa MAHAJAN and More Seema NITIN.

world population is aging at a fast rate and the prevalence of obesity is on the increase, the use of TKA is still in demand. Although the success rates are high in general, patients still complain about residual pain, functional limitations or postoperative dissatisfaction. The correct lining of the limbs and components is always declared to be one of the most decisive factors of the survival and satisfaction in patients with implants (Zambianchi et al. 2021).

Traditionally, postoperative analysis is done in terms of coronal, sagittal and axial planes. It measures the parameters of hip–knee–ankle (HKA) angle, position of the components of the pelvis and legs, and jaw-line orientation and rotation. Malalignments are associated with the distribution of loads, accelerated polyethylene wear, aseptic loosening, instability and premature failure of implants (Hunter et al. 2022). Valid measurement is thus important in the outcome assessment, revision instructions and rehabilitation strategy.

Traditional examination is dependent on plain radiography and computed tomography (CT). Measurements are taken manually by orthopedic surgeons or radiologists. These techniques have the disadvantage of observer dependence, irregular measurements and reduced reproducibility, as well as high workload in high volume conditions (Barbotte et al. 2022). Minor alignment errors can be overlooked, and the conventional methods do not provide much predictive potential for functionality results.

Artificial intelligence (AI) is creating unparalleled possibilities in orthopedic radiography and in postoperative assessment. Deep learning (DL) and machine learning (ML) allow automatic interpretation of images, and feature identification and quantification with great accuracy and stability. AI-assisted systems in TKA have demonstrated positive outcomes in landmark detection, alignment measurement and implant positioning classification, with accuracy equal to that of experts (Bertugli et al. 2024).

In addition to automation, AI systems offer sophisticated analytical services, such as recognition of patterns in the huge data and prediction of outcomes based on multidimensional inputs. Such competencies will be in line with individualized medicine and worth-based orthopedic care. Optimized assessment of alignment with AI has the potential to standardize protocols, minimize human error, and combine alignment data with clinical, functional and biomechanical outcomes (Willemink et al. 2020).

This chapter is an in-depth study of AI-aided postoperative evaluation through the use of AI in TKA-assessed alignment. It includes traditional approaches, AI mechanisms of imaging modalities, validation and performance measures, compatibility with surgical technologies and clinical implications. The problems associated with the quality of data, generalizability, regulatory problems and future research directions are also critically discussed.

3.2. Conventional methods for postoperative alignment assessment after total knee arthroplasty

The measurement of accuracy in postoperative alignment after a TKA is crucial to the evaluation of the preciseness of the surgery, location of the implants and performance of the biomechanics in tasks in the long-run. Traditional methods based on imaging are used in large numbers, but they also have their limitations, which is the reason why AI-assisted approaches are worth considering.

3.2.1. *Plain radiography*

The most popular postoperative alignment assessment tools are standard anteroposterior (AP), lateral and skyline radiographs. HKA radiographs (full length, standing) are considered a gold-standard method of evaluation of coronal limb alignment. The most important parameters are the mechanical axis deviation, anterior tibial positioning and posterior tibial positioning, the coronal positioning of the femur and tibia, the definition of the anterior tibia and posterior tibia slope, and the sagittal flexion of the flexion angle of the femur (Gieroba et al. 2023).

Radiographic evaluation is affordable and widely available. It is, however, dependent on the position of the patient, radiography method and skill of examiners. Misidentification of landmarks could affect the accuracy of measurement by errors of limb rotation, knee flexion contractures and occasional misunderstanding of landmarks (Patel et al. 2022). Manual measurements create inter- and intra-observer errors, particularly in instances where variations are subtle.

3.2.2. *Computed tomography*

A common application of CT is computed tomography (CT), which is used to assess the rotational positioning of (or within) the tibial and femoral components, a procedure that cannot be reliably performed using plain radiography. The CT-based measurements involve measures of rotation of the femur component with reference to the surgical epicondylar axis, and measures of rotation of the tibia component with reference to the tibia tubercles (Skowronek et al. 2021). Extremely close to patellofemoral complications, instability and persistent pain are rotational malalignment.

Although CT has a high spatial resolution and three-dimensional detail, its disadvantages include increased radiation, increased costs, limited availability and time-consuming manual segmentations. CT-based alignment is typically post hoc and does not readily compare with longitudinal outcome monitoring (Han et al. 2021).

3.2.3. *Three-dimensional imaging and EOS systems*

It has been possible to construct three-dimensional images of the lower limb under weight-bearing status with low-dose biplanar radiographic systems, including EOS imaging. The systems enhance precision in global limb positioning and joint positioning, and are less harmful in terms of radiation exposure than CT (Hau et al. 2020). EOS offers concurring appraisal of the coronal, sagittal and axial alignment, which is beneficial in intricate malformations.

The use of EOS is characterized by high costs of installation, limited availability and the requirement to still use manual landmark identification. Measurement variation is also a problem, particularly when metallic implants are involved, which creates imaging artifacts (Klag et al. 2023).

3.2.4. *Observer variability and clinical limitations*

The biggest limitation of traditional assessment of alignment is observer variability. Research demonstrates a significant disparity of measures between surgeons, radiologists and musculoskeletal specialists (Simon et al. 2022). Such discrepancies hamper postoperative care, inter-institutional comparison and multicenter research.

Also, traditional approaches present rigid measurements that are not viewed dynamically to ascertain knee behavior during a walking or stair climbing activity. As a result, radiographic alignment and patient-reported outcomes have insufficient consistency in their correlation (Lawson et al. 2023). The following deficiencies point towards the need for objective and reproducible, data-backed methods.

3.2.5. *Rationale for AI-assisted assessment*

As the volume of TKA increases and outcome optimization is prioritized, the traditional evaluation processes are challenged with regard to scalability and reproducibility. The automation of image analysis, standardization of measurements and additional alignment data with clinical and functional outcomes may be computerized by AI-based assistants (Gurung et al. 2022). The idea of AI-based methods is to reduce the disadvantages of traditional evaluation methods and contribute to the evidence-based decision-making process in knee arthroplasty.

3.3. AI in orthopedic imaging: fundamental concepts

Artificial intelligence has emerged as a potent instrument within the medical imaging field, and is now able to perform analyses, pattern identification and predictive modeling in many fields of orthopedics.

In patients who have received TKA, AI objectively and repeatedly determines the positioning of the implants and the alignment of the limbs in relation to complex images.

3.3.1. *Definitions and scope of AI in orthopedics*

AI is defined as a computing system that simulates functions that are typically done by human intelligence, including the interpretation of images, decision-making and marketing data. Within the orthopedic imaging field,

AI is primarily based on ML and DL of radiographs and CT scans, and three-dimensional reconstructions (D'Angelo et al. 2022).

ML algorithms utilize engineered characteristics acquired from the imaging data, including angles, distances and texture descriptors. Such characteristics are used to train classifiers or regression models, which make predictions about the alignment parameters, or the coding of the implant positioning. At the same time, DL models do not require millions of hand-crafted features since they directly acquire hierarchical features using raw images (Tokgoz et al. 2023).

3.3.2. *DL and convolutional neural networks*

Orthopedic image analysis is mainly dominated by DL and convolutional neural networks (CNNs). CNNs are able to process grid information, including images or excel sheets, identify anatomical landmarks, bone and implant segmentations, and estimate the angle of alignment (Kumar et al. 2026).

CNNs are used in the postoperative evaluation of TKA, detecting important anatomical locations, such as those of the femoral head centers, knee joint centers, tibial plateaus and ankle centers, using long-leg radiographs. The mechanical axis alignment and component orientation can be calculated automatically with these landmarks, and the accuracy of such calculations is equivalent to expert clinicians (Kim et al. 2022).

More complex CNN models such as U-Net and Reset models are frequently used in segmentation and regression. They withstand fluctuations in image quality, patient position and the design of implants, and can hence be implemented at a large clinical scale (Alsinan et al. 2020).

3.3.3. *Supervised, unsupervised and hybrid learning approaches*

AI applications in the field V TKA alignment assessment: supervised learning, in which ground truth is represented by datasets labeled by orthopedic experts, is used in most AI applications in the field. Although supervised models are very accurate, their performance needs large, high quality datasets, and labels that take time and are expensive to generate (Pang et al. 2021).

Unsupervised and semi-supervised learning eliminates the need to have labeled data and discovers inherent patterns within the data of the imaging. Such techniques are also actively being investigated to perform implant clustering, anomaly detection and analysis of alignment deviation in multicenter datasets that have uneven imaging protocols (Raza and Singh 2021).

Hybrid models apply supervised DL with biomechanical constraints in the form of rules, and enhance the interpretability of the models and clinical acceptability. They make sure that AI-generated measurements are based on the orthopedic icons (AbouGrad et al. 2025).

3.3.4. *Performance metrics and validation*

The evaluation measures of AI model performance in alignment assessment commonly include the mean absolute error, intraclass correlation coefficients or Dice similarity coefficients in the case of segmentation, and agreement of the model outcomes with those made by the experts (Goel et al. 2025). Independent datasets improve external validation that is necessary to evaluate inter-institutional/inter-imaging system generalizability.

Recent research demonstrates that AI-aided measurements tend to be less variable than manual measurements, particularly during coronal alignment measurement (van der Graaf et al. 2024). However, strict validation is necessary to promote accuracy in a variety of clinical settings.

3.3.5. *Clinical relevance of AI fundamentals*

This is essential in understanding the AI concepts, and orthopedic surgeons and researchers should carry out a critical evaluation of the performance and limitations of the models. Clear model description, explicability and clinical workflow compatibility are the fundamental attributes of effective research-to-practice translation (Angelov et al. 2021).

The development of AI enables the superior post-traumatic positioning evaluation systems in TKA.

3.4. AI-assisted postoperative alignment assessment techniques after total knee arthroplasty

The methods of postoperative alignment evaluation with the aid of AI in TKA are changing rapidly because of the development and advancement of medical imaging, computational ability and extensive orthopedic databases. These methods aim for automated landmark detection, component segmentation, computing angle of alignment and classification of alignment outliers. AI systems are more efficient, reproducible and scalable than traditional and manual systems.

3.4.1. *Radiograph-based AI alignment assessment*

Plain radiographs are still the most ubiquitous imaging modality used post-TKA, and thus can be a primary focus of AI automation. CNNs and other DL models have been successfully used in long-leg standing radiographs to identify anatomical landmarks that can be used to calculate the alignment. Such landmarks are usually the femur head center, knee joint center, plateau junction of the tibia and ankle joint center.

After being identified, AI systems calculate automatic clinically relevant parameters, including the HKA angle, femur mechanical axis, tibia mechanical axis and alignment of the coronal component. Research studies prove that AI-generated measurements correlate with expert human-generated measurements and tend to emit less inter-observer variation (Shang et al. 2022). This uniformity is especially important when performing high-volume arthroplasty that is characterized by a lack of time to conduct a detailed manual analysis.

Radiographic analysis with the help of AI can also detect subtle malalignment patterns that cannot be seen at first look with human eyes. Early clinical intervention and quality control of surgical practice: automated flagging of alignment outliers allows the analysis of alignment outliers at an early phase.

3.4.2. *AI-based component segmentation and orientation analysis*

In addition to landmark detection, semantic segmentation of the postoperative images into femurs and tibias is carried out using sophisticated models of DL. Segmentation-based technologies allow the accurate estimation of the orientation of the components in relation to the anatomical axes, enhancing the accuracy of measuring the coronal and sagittal positioning.

U-Net-based designs are one of the popular choices in implant segmentation as they maintain the spatial resolution and global context of the object. These models distinguish an imaging artifact between metallic implants and the surrounding bone and soft tissue under the influence of imaging. The variety of measurements on component varus–valgus alignment, anterior tibial slope and the flexion angle of the femur rely on accurate segmentation (Elgarba et al. 2023).

These types of systems minimize the use of manual contour tracing and are found to be particularly useful in longitudinal follow-up studies, in which time-dependent consistency is of great importance.

3.4.3. *CT-based and three-dimensional AI models*

CT is still the criterion upon which rotational alignment can be assessed following TKA. CT is performed by using three-dimensional CNNs, where AI assists in the automatic localization of the tibial and femoral components, and locating the axes of rotation.

The rotation of the femoral component in reference to the surgical epicondylar axis and tibial rotation in reference to the tibial tubercle can be estimated with high accuracy by learning the AI models on volumetric CT data. AI analysis cost, compared to manual CT measurements, reduces the processing time by many times; it is also accurate or even better (Yang and Qian 2025).

The possibility of virtual reconstruction of postoperative alignment of limbs by three-dimensional AI models can also be carried out, and the evaluation of limb position in the coronal, sagittal and axial planes. Such reconstructions give insight into complicated malalignment patterns that could lead to patients being dissatisfied or implants failing.

3.4.4. *Integration with navigation and robotic systems*

Computer-assisted navigation and robotized TKA platforms are being combined with AI and aligned evaluation more often. Analysis of AI during post-operation is comparable to intraoperative data concerning alignment to assess the accuracy of surgical operations and determine their deviation sources.

Other new systems apply AI-based feedback loops, with postsurgical alignment information improving preoperative planning systems and execution plans. The framework of continuous improvement of precision in surgery and predictability of outcomes uses this closed-loop structure (Singh and Patel 2024).

3.4.5. *Predictive and outcome-oriented AI models*

In addition to descriptive assessment, AI systems are being designed to forecast clinical outcomes, using postoperative alignment information. ML models used to resolve alignment parameters and apply them together with demographic, biomechanical and functional outcome measures determine the alignment thresholds linked to patient satisfaction and implant longevity at the optimum level.

These prediction models do not follow the conventional paradigm of neutral mechanical alignment, but uphold more novel ideas such as kinematic and functional alignment strategies. In the long term, AI analysis facilitates an assessment of the relationship between the results and alignment of its magnitude that was once unfeasible to complete manually (Tolk et al. 2020).

3.4.6. *Clinical impact and advantages*

All in all, AI-based postoperative alignment assessment has numerous benefits compared to traditional methods, such as decelerated observer variability, quicker analysis and superior integration of data. These advantages make AI a helpful clinical decision-support tool in contemporary knee arthroplasty practice, as it has the potential to enhance the short- and long-term outcomes.

The comparison of traditional and AI-enabled postoperative alignment assessment methodology with TKA is presented in Table 3.1.

Assessment aspect	Conventional methods	AI-assisted methods	Clinical advantage of AI
Imaging modalities	Plain radiographs, CT, EOS	Radiographs, CT, EOS with AI automation	Uses existing imaging without additional burden
Landmark identification	Manual, observer dependent	Automated landmark detection (CNN-based)	Reduced inter- and intra-observer variability
Coronal alignment (HKA angle)	Manual angle measurement	Automated calculation with high agreement	Improved reproducibility and efficiency
Sagittal component alignment	Manual estimation	AI-based component segmentation and orientation analysis	Greater precision in component positioning
Rotational alignment	Manual CT measurements	AI-driven 3D CT analysis	Faster and more accurate rotational assessment
Time efficiency	Time-consuming	Rapid, automated processing	Reduced clinician workload
Reproducibility	Moderate, operator dependent	High, standardized outputs	Consistency across centers
Outcome prediction	Limited	AI models linking alignment to functional outcomes	Supports personalized alignment strategies
Workflow integration	Stand-alone assessment	PACS/navigation/robotic system integration	Seamless clinical decision support

Table 3.1. *Comparison of conventional and AI-assisted postoperative alignment assessment methods after total knee arthroplasty*

3.5. Clinical validation and comparative effectiveness of AI-assisted alignment assessment

Tasks: AI-assisted postoperative alignment assessment after TKA should be adopted by the clinic on the condition of strict validation and evidence that it is safer or, at least, equally effective. In recent years, AI alignment tools have been tested by numerous studies on historic and new clinical data.

3.5.1. *Validation against expert measurements*

The evaluation of the majority of AI systems is based on a comparison with ground-truth annotations of a set of seasoned orthopedic surgeons or musculoskeletal radiologists. Validation will typically give intraclass correlation coefficients, mean absolute error and Bland–Altman limits. These analyses demonstrate a very high consensus in terms of the alignment of the corula, particularly, the HKA angle and the component varus–valgus orientation.

In some of the studies, the AI measurements were less varied than manual measurements, especially in cases where the alignment was close to the threshold limits. Minimizing observer error is important in clinical terms, as any difference will affect the lifespan of implants. The strength of AI is also evident in its ability to be similar among various designs of implants and imaging procedures as well.

3.5.2. *Time efficiency and workflow integration*

In addition to accuracy, AI contributes to a lot of efficiency. Assessment may require several minutes when manually conducted, particularly in busy arthroplasty centers. AI can handle X-rays or CT scans in seconds and therefore reduces clinician workload significantly.

Such speed is used in the routine checks of all TKA patients rather than selective tests. Introducing AI to picture archiving and communication systems, as well as electronic health records, additionally facilitates the workflow, allowing surgeons to check metrics in visits following the surgery.

3.5.3. *Correlation with clinical outcomes*

One of the main validation points is the relationship of AI-generated alignment and patient outcomes. According to recent research, AI measurements have been associated with pain measurements, functional tests and implant survival.

Massive AI scans have shown maximum alignment to different people and suggest the substitution of inflexible goals with individual strategies. So, AI does not only enhance the precision of the measurement, but the knowledge of the biomechanics post-TKA.

3.5.4. *Comparative effectiveness versus conventional methods*

AI systems have comparable or even greater accuracy, and significantly greater reproducibility compared to manual assessment. AI models based on CT, especially, prove to be more successful than manual methods in rotational alignment, which has traditionally been a problematic area.

Nonetheless, the literature also makes us remember that AI is not something that can substitute clinical judgment, but is a decision-support tool. Even now, surgeons have to comprehend alignment data in relation to the anatomy, symptoms and objectives of each patient.

3.5.5. *Multicenter and external validation*

Generalizability is necessary through external checks by various institutions. Multicenter trials indicate that AI evaluation does not compromise on performance on patients and the imaging settings of various groups. Continuous validation should be used to solve dataset composition and implant producer bias.

3.6. Challenges, limitations and ethical considerations

Although this has been achieved, AI-aid postoperative alignment assessment is an area that demands to be overcome before it becomes common.

3.6.1. *Data quality and bias*

The quality and variety of data are very important to the AI models. The bias of models using under-representation of particular demographics, type of implant or type of imaging may restrict generalizability. It requires large and multicenter datasets that have standardized annotation protocols.

3.6.2. *Interpretability and clinical trust*

A lot of DL models are black boxes, which do not provide much information about measurement mechanisms. Such obscurity may compromise the trust of clinicians.

It is essential to increase the level of transparency with the help of landmark visualizations and confidence scores.

3.6.3. *Regulatory and legal considerations*

AI medical machines should adhere to safety, efficacy and data-privacy laws. Attention can also delay execution, depending on the location. Besides, there is no clarity about AI-directed decisions in terms of legal responsibility.

3.6.4. *Cost and infrastructure requirements*

Although AI may reduce long-term costs with efficiency, the upfront software, hardware and training expenses may be high. Limited resources are settings that may find it difficult to implement AI evaluation unless there is an adequate infrastructure.

3.6.5. *Ethical and privacy concerns*

Big imaging datasets pose a security hazard to privacy. The ethical use of AI also requires compliance with the laws on data protection and keeping patients' trust.

3.7. Future directions and emerging trends

The development of AI, data fusion and individualized treatment lays the foundation of the future of postoperative alignment evaluation following TKA.

3.7.1. *Personalized alignment strategies*

AI analysis allows the creation of personalized targets of alignment depending on anatomy, gait and functional needs. This individualistic method is to enhance satisfaction and long-term results compared to one-size-fits-all techniques.

3.7.2. *Integration with wearable and functional data*

The integration of AI alignment measurement and wearable sensor data and gait analysis is a new area of research. This integration may provide dynamic knee information compared to inactive imaging.

3.7.3. *Continuous learning systems*

The next-generation AI platforms can include ongoing learning, and the models can be updated with new incoming information. This flexibility will lead to future performance and favor changes in the surgical practices.

3.7.4. *Role in revision arthroplasty*

Failure mechanisms can also be detected with the aid of AI-assessed testing and used to plan the revision of TKA. Malalignment patterns that are automated help to intervene early and improve revision processes.

3.8. Conclusion

Correct postoperative positioning is critical in TKA. Conventional imaging-based techniques offer a platform, yet they have low reproducibility, efficiency and predictions of results. The reverse is true of AI-assessed evaluation, which provides automated, objective and scalable solutions. It has always been able to measure alignment correctly across modalities, and provides the opportunity to analyze the relationship between alignment and outcomes at a large scale. AI allows the integration of clinical and functional measurements with alignment measures, which can lead to individualized, data-driven arthroplasty care. Despite its existing limitations, especially related to the quality of data, its comprehensibility and regulation, AI methods are being optimized in on-going research. There is an opportunity to make post-operative assessment much more transparent and involved in clinical systems, which is why AI can change all of this and increase patient satisfaction, as well as enhance the long-term outcomes following TKA.

3.9. References

AbouGrad, H., Yegamati, M., Mather, M. (2025). Hybrid deep learning healthcare AI framework for real-time human pose estimation and remote patient monitoring to support TKR physiotherapy. In *14th International Conference on Human Interaction and Emerging Technologies: Artificial Intelligence & Future Applications, IHIET-FS 2025*, 10–12 June, University of East London, London, 134–144. AHFE International.

Alsinan, A.Z., Patel, V.M., Hacihaliloglu, I. (2020). Bone shadow segmentation from ultrasound data for orthopedic surgery using GAN. *International Journal of Computer Assisted Radiology and Surgery*, 15(9), 1477–1485.

Angelov, P.P., Soares, E.A., Jiang, R., Arnold, N.I., Atkinson, P.M. (2021). Explainable artificial intelligence: An analytical review. *Wiley Interdisciplinary Reviews: Data Mining and Knowledge Discovery*, 11(5), e1424.

Barbotte, F., Delord, M., Pujol, N. (2022). Coronal knee alignment measurements differ on long-standing radiographs vs. by navigation. *Orthopaedics & Traumatology: Surgery & Research*, 108(5), 103112.

Bertugli, E., Lustig, S., Parratte, S., Catani, F., Batailler, C. (2024). Artificial intelligence in knee arthroplasty. In *Artificial Intelligence in Orthopaedic Surgery Made Easy*, Familiari, F., Galasso, O., Gasparini, G. (eds). Springer, Cham, 55–63.

D'Angelo, T., Caudo, D., Blandino, A., Albrecht, M.H., Vogl, T.J., Gruenewald, L.D., Gaeta, M., Yel, I., Koch, V., Martin, S.S. et al. (2022). Artificial intelligence, machine learning and deep learning in musculoskeletal imaging: Current applications. *Journal of Clinical Ultrasound*, 50(9), 1414–1431.

Elgarba, B.M., Van Aelst, S., Swaity, A., Morgan, N., Shujaat, S., Jacobs, R. (2023). Deep learning-based segmentation of dental implants on cone-beam computed tomography images: A validation study. *Journal of Dentistry*, 137, 104639.

Gieroba, T.J., Marasco, S., Babazadeh, S., Di Bella, C., van Bavel, D. (2023). Arithmetic hip knee angle measurement on long leg radiograph versus computed tomography—inter-observer and intra-observer reliability. *Arthroplasty*, 5(1), 35.

Goel, A., Singhal, A., Kumar, S. (2025). Assessment of AI models in healthcare: Performance metrics and applications across critical diseases. *International Journal of System Assurance Engineering and Management*, 1–9. doi: 10.1007/s13198-025-02968-1.

van der Graaf, J.W., van Hooff, M.L., van Ginneken, B., Huisman, M., Rutten, M., Lamers, D., Lessmann, N., de Kleuver, M. (2024). Development and validation of AI-based automatic measurement of coronal Cobb angles in degenerative scoliosis using sagittal lumbar MRI. *European Radiology*, 34(9), 5748–5757.

Gurung, B., Liu, P., Harris, P.D., Sagi, A., Field, R.E., Sochart, D.H., Tucker, K., Asopa, V. (2022). Artificial intelligence for image analysis in total hip and total knee arthroplasty: A scoping review. *The Bone & Joint Journal*, 104(8), 929–937.

Han, C., Liu, J., Wu, Y., Chong, Y., Chai, X., Weng, X. (2021). To predict the length of hospital stay after total knee arthroplasty in an orthopedic center in China: The use of machine learning algorithms. *Frontiers in Surgery*, 8, 606038.

Hau, M.Y., Menon, D.K., Chan, R.J., Chung, K.Y., Chau, W.W., Ho, K.W. (2020). Two-dimensional/three-dimensional EOS™ imaging is reliable and comparable to traditional X-ray imaging assessment of knee osteoarthritis aiding surgical management. *The Knee*, 27(3), 970–979.

Hunter, C.W., Deer, T.R., Jones, M.R., Chang Chien, G.C., D'Souza, R.S., Davis, T., Eldon, E.R., Esposito, M.F., Goree, J.H., Hewan-Lowe, L. et al. (2022). Consensus guidelines on interventional therapies for knee pain (STEP Guidelines) from the American Society of Pain and Neuroscience. *Journal of Pain Research*, 15, 2683–2745. doi: 10.2147/JPR.S370469.

Kim, B., Lee, D.W., Lee, S., Ko, S., Jo, C., Park, J., Choi, B.S., Krych, A.J., Pareek, A., Han, H.S. et al. (2022). Automated detection of surgical implants on plain knee radiographs using a deep learning algorithm. *Medicina*, 58(11), 1677.

Klag, E.A., Lizzio, V.A., Charters, M.A., Ayoola, A.S., Wesemann, L., Banka, T.R., North, W.T. (2023). Increased accuracy in templating for total knee arthroplasty using 3D models generated from radiographs. *The Journal of Knee Surgery*, 36(08), 837–842.

Kumar, A., Batta, P., Ahuja, S., Rathore, P.S. (eds) (2026). *AI-driven Innovations in Physiotherapy and Oncology 1*. ISTE Ltd, London and Wiley, Hoboken, NJ.

Lawson, A., Naylor, J., Mittal, R., Kale, M., Xuan, W., Harris, I.A. (2023). Does radiographic alignment correlate with patient-reported functional outcomes and posttreatment complications in older patients treated for wrist fractures? *The Journal of Hand Surgery*, 48(6), 533–543.

Pang, T., Wong, J.H., Ng, W.L., Chan, C.S. (2021). Semi-supervised GAN-based radiomics model for data augmentation in breast ultrasound mass classification. *Computer Methods and Programs in Biomedicine*, 203, 106018.

Patel, D.V., Dávila Castrodad, I.M., Kurowicki, J., McInerney, V.K. and Scillia, A.J. (2022). Patellofemoral instability. In *Arthroscopy*, Suarez-Ahedo, C. (ed.). IntechOpen, London. doi: 10.5772/intechopen.94681.

Raza, K. and Singh, N.K. (2021). A tour of unsupervised deep learning for medical image analysis. *Current Medical Imaging Reviews*, 17(9), 1059–1077.

Shang, G., Hu, M., Guo, J., Hao, X., Xiang, S. (2022). Using short knee radiographs to predict the coronal alignment after TKA: Is it an accurate proxy for HKA on full-length images? *Journal of Orthopaedic Surgery and Research*, 17(1), 340.

Simon, S., Schwarz, G.M., Aichmair, A., Frank, B.J., Hummer, A., DiFranco, M.D., Dominkus, M., Hofstaetter, J.G. (2022). Fully automated deep learning for knee alignment assessment in lower extremity radiographs: A cross-sectional diagnostic study. *Skeletal Radiology*, 51(6), 1249–1259.

Singh, J. and Patel, P. (2024). Robotics in arthroplasty: Historical progression, contemporary applications, and future horizons with artificial intelligence (AI) integration. *Cureus*, 16(8), e67611. doi: 10.7759/cureus.67611.

Skowronek, P., Arnold, M., Starke, C., Bartyzel, A., Moser, L.B., Hirschmann, M.T., European Knee Associates (EKA) (2021). Intra-and postoperative assessment of femoral component rotation in total knee arthroplasty: An EKA knee expert group clinical review. *Knee Surgery, Sports Traumatology, Arthroscopy*, 29(3), 772–782.

Tokgoz, E., Levitt, S., Sosa, D., Carola, N.A., Patel, V. (eds) (2023). Artificial intelligence, deep learning, and machine learning applications in total knee arthroplasty. In *Total Knee Arthroplasty: A Review of Medical and Biomedical Engineering and Science Concepts*. Springer, Cham, 215–245.

Tolk, J.J., Waarsing, J.E., Janssen, R.P., van Steenbergen, L.N., Bierma-Zeinstra, S.M., Reijman, M. (2020). Development of preoperative prediction models for pain and functional outcome after total knee arthroplasty using the Dutch arthroplasty register data. *The Journal of Arthroplasty*, 35(3), 690–698.

Willemink, M.J., Koszek, W.A., Hardell, C., Wu, J., Fleischmann, D., Harvey, H., Folio, L.R., Summers, R.M., Rubin, D.L., Lungren, M.P. (2020). Preparing medical imaging data for machine learning. *Radiology*, 295(1), 4–15.

Yang, T.J. and Qian, W. (2025). AI-assisted 3D planning of CT parameters for personalized femoral prosthesis selection in total hip arthroplasty. *Therapeutics and Clinical Risk Management*, 21, 905–916. doi: 10.2147/TCRM.S521755.

Zambianchi, F., Bazzan, G., Marcovigi, A., Pavesi, M., Illuminati, A., Ensini, A., Catani, F. (2021). Joint line is restored in robotic-arm-assisted total knee arthroplasty performed with a tibia-based functional alignment. *Archives of Orthopaedic and Trauma Surgery*, 141(12), 2175–2184.

4

Functional Outcome Prediction Following Open Tibial Fractures Using AI-Based Models

Open tibial fractures are severe wounds in the long bones. They tend to be followed by a lot of soft-tissue damage, high risk of infection, retarded healing and permanent functional issues. Many clinical inferences depend on numerous interacting factors: the severity of the injury, patient characteristics and the nature of dealing with the injury to predict the extent of successful recovery of patients are major clinical challenges. The prognostic models and scoring systems that exist are usually not very accurate and generalized. In the recent past, artificial intelligence (AI) models have proved to be promising. AI has the potential to enhance outcome prediction by dealing with high-dimensional and complicated clinical data. This chapter evaluates the latest conditions of AI methodologies in forecasting the outcomes of surgery after open tibial fractures, focusing on machine learning and deep learning methods, datasets, feature-selection guides and performance measures presented in the literature. It also addresses the benefits of AI compared to traditional statistics – improved accuracy, flexibility and real-time clinical usefulness – and critically evaluates the impediments, including the data quality, interpretations, bias and clinical integration. The problem of AI in orthopedic trauma care in terms of ethical and regulatory considerations is discussed. The synthesis of the current evidence shows that AI-based predictive models can be used to inform personal treatment, optimize the rehabilitation process and enhance shared decision-making in patients with open tibial fractures, which the chapter illustrates. It suggests future research directions and implementation steps that help to make AI translation into the everyday orthopedic practice responsible.

4.1. Introduction

The cause of open tibial fracture is orthopedic trauma that is difficult to cure. The tibia is encountered directly beneath the skin and is somewhat

Chapter written by Amol S. DHAWALE and Dalavi Surekha GORAKH.

covered by soft tissue, and is also extremely vulnerable to contamination. These injuries are normally due to high-energy accidents such as road-traffic accidents, industrial accidents or even falls from a height. They induce great bone and soft-tissue damage. However, even after the evolution of surgery fixation, soft-tissue reconstruction and infection control, patients have long-term recovery and significant functional impairment.

The functional recovery following open fracture of the tibia relies on numerous factors: severity/extent of the fracture, soft-tissue damage, comorbidities in patients, timing of administration, fixation methods, rehabilitation regimen and postoperative events. Outcome measures are used by clinicians to determine physical function, pain, mobility and quality of life, including the Lower Extremity Functional Scale (LEFS), Short Form-36 (SF-36), American Orthopedic Foot and Ankle Society (AOFAS) score and EuroQol-5D (EQ-5D). Nonetheless, the problem of long-term recovery with traditional clinical judgment or the conventional scoring system is still inaccurate.

Conventional prediction instruments, such as the Gustilo Anderson classification and the Mangled Extremity Severity Score (MESS), were not intended to predict functional outcome, and appear to be less accurate in the contemporary patient groups. This has led to increasing attention on AI-based models, in particular, machine learning (ML) and deep learning (DL) algorithms, which are capable of learning complex nonlinear dependencies from large amounts of data and enhancing the prediction of outcomes for individuals (Tian et al. 2024).

The chapter summarizes existing data on AI models to predict functional results following an open tibial fracture. It puts their procedures, effect, clinical significance and potential into the limelight.

4.2. Clinical significance of open tibial fractures

Open tibia fractures are one of the most significant orthopedic trauma injuries as they occur frequently, are serious and can significantly impact the functionality of the patient and overall life quality. The tibia is located directly underneath the skin on the inner-frontal side of the leg, and hence, it

is particularly prone to be revealed when a high-energy injury takes place. Therefore, such fractures typically imply a big scope of devastated soft tissues, contamination and lack of blood supply; as a result, treatment is complicated, and the final results are unpredictable.

Epidemiology reveals that road-traffic crashes, workplace accidents and falls from a height are the greatest causes that affect people of working age, who are still young (Nicolaides et al. 2021). This trend only magnifies the social and economic effects, because long-term recovery and a non-productive status may result in prolonged absence of activity, loss of revenue and lower productivity overall. Direct costs will be comprised of the surgery, hospital stay and rehabilitation, whereas the indirect costs will be the long-term disability and psychosocial problems.

An open tibial fracture is a condition that is clinically treated using numerous resources and multidisciplinary approaches. Short-term objectives include cleaning the wound, stabilizing the bone, preventing infection and covering the soft tissue. Although modern fixation and reconstructive measures are used, complications are still prevalent. Any infection, retardation, nonunion and chronic bone infection may postpone recovery and may need additional surgery and prolonged recovery, that will cause even more stress, both physically and emotionally (Cortez et al. 2022).

Delayed healing is not the only functional post-open tibial fracture issue. Patients may experience persistent pain, muscular weakness, rigid stiff joints, abnormal gait and trouble in performing their daily tasks. Instances of minimal soft tissues and distal tibial fractures typically result in limited movement in the ankle and knee. Even many years after injury, these deficits are manifested in poorer scores in the Lower Extremity Functional Scale (LEFS) and American Orthopaedic Foot and Ankle Society (AOFAS) score (Cortez et al. 2022).

The level of quality of life also becomes significantly lower. There are prospective changes in the scores of physical health, with the Short Form-36 (SF-36) and EuroQol-5D (EQ-5D) indicating permanent reductions relative to actually occurring age scores (Ochen et al. 2020). It also has the tendency to impact mental health, particularly among individuals who have chronic pain or slow healing, or even individuals who take too long to heal but continue to work. Such results alert us to assess the physical and psychosocial recovery.

One of the major indicators of functional recovery and social reintegration is the ability to return to work. Extreme open tibial fractures tend to result in prolonged job loss, more so in physically demanding jobs. Late or incomplete return to employment is associated with a high Gustilo Anderson grade, postoperative complications, continued pain and poor early function scores, which are related to financial stress, diminished confidence and quality of life.

The recovery process is hard to predict as there are numerous factors which affect functional recovery. The severity of injury scales and clinician judgment can only provide a slight idea about long-term functioning. The diversity of patient age, pattern of injury, procedure and compliance in rehab result in a large variation in the outcome, irrespective of the similarity in the fracture grade among the patients. This ambiguity makes patient counseling, rehab planning and allocation of resources more difficult (Schade et al. 2021).

Therefore, open tibial fractures are not only important in the operating room, but also in long-term functionality and quality of life. Personalized care presupposes effective prediction of outcomes, rehabilitation requirements and chances of a return to work. AI programs can assist in integrating clinical data and patient reports to make predictions about individual outcomes, which could lead to more effective expectations and tailored rehab, and lessen the burden over the long term.

4.3. Traditional approaches to outcome prediction

The outcome prediction tools mainly used in the past depended on the experience of clinicians, injury classifications and simple-mode statistics. These methods are only useful when there is a need to make an immediate decision, but not in the long-run functionality. Most traditional models are outgrown by the complexity of open tibial fractures, which entail damage to the bones, soft tissues, biology of the patient and factors of rehab.

Still, the Gustilo Anderson system remains in use as a classification system of open fractures, based on the size of the wounds, contamination and soft-tissue destruction. It assists in forecasting the risk of infection and use of antibiotics and surgery, but not functional recovery. It is loosely correlated with patient-reported outcome measures (PROM) such as LEFS and SF-36 scores, and interobserver reliability has low validity (Kumar et al. 2025).

Other scores such as the Mangled Extremity Severity Score, Predictive Salvage Index and Limb Salvage Index were simply created to determine the choice between limb salvage and amputation. They pay attention to the ischemia time, vascular injuries and shock, and fail to embrace rehabilitation potential, motivation and long-term quality of life. They can therefore only be of limited use in predicting an independent functioning or a return to work (Nayar et al. 2022).

Age, fracture severity, infection, delayed union and smoking have been predicted as the conventional statistical techniques that multivariate linear or logistic regressions have identified.

Nevertheless, these models presuppose linear correlation, independent predictors and constant variables, which are hardly similar to nonlinear functional recovery (Lorente et al. 2024).

Lastly, most conventional models refer to the use of fixed data points where the changes in patients across time in rehab are not taken into consideration. The dynamics of open tibial fracture recovery are always dynamic and will change several months and years later due to the dynamic changes in clinical and psychosocial factors. Therefore, such traditional methods tend to have low predictive validity and low external validity in different groups of patients.

4.4. Overview of artificial intelligence in orthopedic trauma

Artificial intelligence has become one of the most prominent tools in orthopedic trauma because it offers analytical features with capabilities that are above those of traditional statistics. AI is used to describe a set of computer systems, which are able to execute tasks that should apply human intelligence, including pattern recognition functions, decision-making processes and predictive analytics. AI in orthopedic trauma is used in the detection of fractures, surgical planning, evaluation of complication risks and functional outcome prediction (Misir and Yuce 2025).

ML is a fundamental attribute of AI allowing the algorithms to learn and improve without any special programming. Labeled datasets based on supervised learning are particularly handy when predicting outcomes such as functional scores, rehabilitation periods and return to work. Unsupervised learning assists in the discovery of undetected patterns or patient sub-groups in large datasets of trauma. It has a more advanced form, known as DL, which involves medical images and longitudinal clinical records, and operates on the basis of multilayer neural networks to process high-dimensional data (Fritz et al. 2023).

The promise of AI in orthopedic trauma is in the possibility to combine heterogeneous sources of data. The determination of functional outcomes following open tibia fracture involves the assessment of demographics, injury characteristics, surgical variables, rehabilitation measurements and the patient-reported outcome. Artificial intelligence models have the ability to embrace nonlinear, intricate interactions between these variables so that their modeling forecasts are more precise and personalized than the conventional models (Saccomanno et al. 2024).

Now, AI is being used increasingly as large-scale trauma registries, digital rehabilitation monitoring systems and electronic health records become commonplace. Such data will give the quantity and diversity required to develop powerful artificial intelligence models that can be generalized to patient groups and clinical environments. Artificial intelligence will be able to constantly adapt to new information, forecasting changes whenever treatment regimens and rehabilitation models are changed.

4.5. ML techniques for functional outcome prediction

The AI-based functional outcome prediction models on orthopedic trauma rely on ML. These are methods involving the analysis of complex datasets in order to establish patterns and relationships that may not be visible using conventional methods. When it comes to open tibial fractures,

ML is used to predict the LEFS increase, SF-36 physical functioning scores, time period of rehabilitation and return to work.

The most prevalent outcome predictive supervised learning models are as follows. Decision trees, random forests, gradient-boosting machines and support vector machines are some of the algorithms that are trained using labeled data. Random forests and gradient-boosting models are both specifically applicable to clinical data since they can handle missing data and nonlinear interaction with each other, which is more accurate than the traditional regression models (Shi et al. 2023).

Orthopedic prediction of outcome is another area of the support vector machine technology, particularly with smaller datasets. SVMs categorize patient recovery as satisfactory or unsatisfactory by constructing the best boundaries of decision in high-dimensional space. Nonetheless, they are not as interpretable as they can be a challenge to clinical adoption (Tared et al. 2024).

DL models such as artificial neural networks are characterized by their ability to process high-dimensional data of complex nature. Convolutional neural networks are used to analyze radiography features associated with fracture healing and alignment, which are correlated with outcomes. Recurrent neural networks and LSTM networks capture the depiction of the temporal recovery patterns, including gradual increases of the LEFS score over the serial visits (Shaikh et al. 2024; Cui 2024).

Accuracy, AUC and error are used to measure model performance. Research findings consistently show that ML models perform better than traditional statistical methods, particularly when longitudinal and rehabilitation data are taken into consideration (Peng et al. 2023). These data point to the ability of ML to improve functional outcome prediction and provide patients with open tibial fracture with personalized care pathways.

4.6. Data sources and feature engineering

4.6.1. *Clinical and demographic variables*

The significant predictors in AI-based predictive models are the age of a patient, sex, body weight index, smoking status, diabetes and the mechanism of injury. These variables are similar in that they are always linked to delayed recovery and low functional scores after open tibia fractures (Tian et al. 2020).

4.6.2. *Injury and surgical characteristics*

There are injury-specific characteristics (Grade Gustilo–Anderson, fracture pattern, contamination and injury to vascularity) and vital inputs. Surgery factors such as fixation mode, soft-tissue coverage time and frequency play an important role in functional recovery and duration of rehabilitation (You and Schneider 2020).

4.6.3. *Rehabilitation and return-to-work parameters*

Variables revolving around rehabilitation are central to the prediction of functional outcome. They comprise time to weight-bearing, compliance with physiotherapy, retraining of the range-of-motion and recovery of muscle strength. The use of rehabilitation data enhances the accuracy of existing AI models when predicting LEFS improvement and time to return to work (Kokkotis et al. 2022).

Return-to-work outcomes have become the most popular indicator of functional recovery. This is through AI models which classify patients who face the risk of long-term absence from the workforce depending on the severity of injury, workplace demands and initial functional ratings. These speculations justify vocational rehabilitation planning and strategies of employer engagement (Duong et al. 2020).

4.7. Patient-reported outcome measures in AI-based prediction models

Patient-reported outcome measures (PROMs) are useful in evaluating postoperative recovery of open tibial fracture. They are indicators of the patients' perception of quality of life, mobility and pain. The Lower Extremity Functional Scale (LEFS), Short Form-36 (SF-36), American Orthopaedic Foot and Ankle Society (AOFAS) score and EuroQol-5D are the most available PROMs. The measures have become targets and input data for AI models.

LEFS is a particularly effective tool to assess the function of lower limbs and supports the identification of minor shifts in rehabilitation. AI can predict long-term recovery by preoperative LEFS and identify patients who are disabled (Zhang et al. 2025). The SF-36 physical component provides a general picture of health-related quality of life and regularly serves as the result variable in prognostic models.

Despite it being a part of clinician-reported data, the AOFAS score continues to be relevant in the evaluation of the functioning of the ankle and hindfoot after distal tibia fracture.

In cases where AI is implemented together with AOFAS sub-scores, the scores are more likely to differentiate between satisfactory and poor performance as opposed to traditional scoring (Schurz et al. 2023).

The AI models based on PROMs introduce patient-centered information in clinical practice. Monitoring PROMs over a certain time, AI will be able to identify small tendencies and determine when the recovery will take a wrong turn, taking timely measures.

4.8. Prediction of rehabilitation trajectories and return to work

Postoperative treatment following open tibial fractures is time-consuming and accordingly, resource-consuming, and recovery varies significantly across patients. The progress can be predicted by AI, duration of rehabilitation and milestones such as walking and returning to work. These are lessons used to tailor physiotherapy and establish attainable objectives.

ML models which operate on early postoperative data and adherence measures of the rehab can precisely forecast when patients will attain such milestones as full weight-bearing and non-assisted walking (Lokerman et al. 2023). With the inclusion of attendance during physiotherapy, improvement of range-of-motion and strength tests, AI can constantly predict recovery.

One of the outcomes is predicting return to work due to its socioeconomic impact. A high Gustilo grade, physically demanding jobs, continued pain and low early LEFS scores are also known to predict delays in AI classification models (Agarwal et al. 2023). Such AI models are more effective at dividing patients into risk groups as opposed to simple regression.

AI predictions aid in organizing multidisciplinary rehab by identifying patients that require additional physiotherapy, mental health help or vocational rehabilitation. They also contribute to joint decision-making, through the provision of individual recovery schedules and prognoses.

4.9. Comparison of AI-based models with traditional predictive methods

Comparative studies on AI models and traditional statistics report that AI outperforms the traditional ones. Regular regression is based on linearity and independent variables, which fail to reflect the complicated connections that influence recovery in the aftermath of open tibial fractures.

Random forest and gradient-based boosting outperform logistic regression in terms of predicting bad outcomes of LEFS and SF-36, having high AUCs and reduced errors (Marra 2024).

DL introduces one more level of accuracy in the form of time-series data and imaging, which provide a more precise image of recovery.

A key advantage of AI is that it is flexible. In comparison to fixed traditional models, AI is retrained using new data, so, it can be used more generally across populations and settings. This comes in handy, particularly in orthopedic trauma, where the protocols and rehab plans keep changing (Guo et al. 2024).

Although AI works better than that, it also has some problems with interpretability and its acceptance. It is essential to use explainable AI approaches to bring transparency and enhance clinical trust.

Table 4.1 interprets the results of traditional and AI-based methods for functional outcome prediction following open tibial fracture.

Aspect	Traditional predictive approaches	AI-based predictive models
Primary purpose	Injury severity classification, limb salvage decision-making	Prediction of long-term functional recovery and rehabilitation outcomes
Common tools	Gustilo–Anderson classification, MESS, clinician judgment	Machine learning (RF, GBM, SVM), deep learning (ANN, CNN, RNN-LSTM)
Data handling	Limited variables, linear assumptions	High-dimensional, nonlinear, multimodal data integration
Data sources	Injury characteristics, basic clinical variables	Clinical, surgical, rehabilitation, PROMs, imaging, longitudinal data
Functional outcomes predicted	Not specifically designed for functional outcomes	LEFS, SF-36, AOFAS, EQ-5D, return to work
Temporal modeling	Static, single-time-point analysis	Dynamic, longitudinal outcome forecasting
Predictive accuracy	Limited, poor generalizability	Superior accuracy and adaptability across populations
Clinical utility	Acute decision support	Personalized rehabilitation planning and shared decision-making
Limitations	Poor functional correlation, interobserver variability	Interpretability, data quality, ethical and regulatory challenges

Table 4.1. *Comparison of traditional and AI-based approaches for functional outcome prediction after open tibial fractures*

4.10. Clinical applications of AI-based functional outcome prediction

Functional outcome prediction models built using AI can improve the treatment of patients with open tibial fractures by improving individualized, data-driven decision-making during treatment. One of the applications is early-risk stratification: AI identifies the patients in accordance with the estimated risk of achieving functional recovery criteria in the form of LEFS, SF-36 or AOFAS scores. Early detection of high-risk individuals allows clinicians to implement proactive strategies earlier – more vigorous rehabilitation, better follow-up or referral to multidisciplinary care groups sooner (Beaulieu-Jones et al. 2021).

In surgery planning, AI will predict the functionality of the various fixation techniques, soft-tissue coverage schedules and weight-bearing timelines. The models generate personal predictions of outcome by incorporating the severity of injuries, comorbidities and procedure details supporting the shared decision-making. This assists clinicians in establishing realistic recovery projections, describing possible shortcomings and predicting work establishment.

The other important application is rehabilitation optimization. Longitudinal functional tracking AI is predictive of rehabilitation trends, and it identifies those who deviate off course. Clinicians and the physiotherapist can then make adjustments related to the intensity, duration and areas of focus in real time, thus improving efficiency and reducing wastage. The data provided by wearables and digital physiotherapy platforms are more continuous, which means that these predictions can be increased.

Return-to-work prediction has become an issue of concern for open tibial fracture patients. AI categorizes patients based on the probability of returning to employment prior to the injury and takes job demands, first functional ratings and psychosocial factors into account. Such insights help in early vocational rehabilitation planning and persuading employers to reduce absences at work and socioeconomic burden (Cirillo et al. 2025).

4.11. Challenges and limitations of AI-based models

In spite of favorable outcomes, the use of AI outcome models in orthopedic trauma faces a number of obstacles which hinder its adoption. The issues of data quality and completeness are still significant. Incidentally, clinical records are filled with responding gaps, inconsistency and different timings to assess outcomes. LEFS and SF-36 are not extensively gathered regularly as PROMs, which restricts the model training and limits the generalizability.

The second challenge is the interpretability of a model. High-performance AI, specifically DL, may serve as a black box, as it provides answers without explaining factors that lead to the answer. This clouding may result in lack of clinician trust and acceptance. The inclusion of explainable AI, which is feature-importance analysis and visualization, will make the predictions meaningfully clinical and ethically defendable (Jasen 2025).

Prejudice and impartiality are also severe problems. Models which have been trained on samples without certain groups that are not represented in the sample, such as patients, manual workers, low-socioeconomic employees, etc., may lead to false or unfair predictions, exacerbating healthcare inequality. Biases need to be reduced by conducting rigorous external validation in varied populations.

The integration of AI tools into the current electronic health record systems would necessitate a large-scale technical infrastructure, standards of interoperability and training of clinicians. Trauma environments are busy, which introduces time limitations and can leave clinicians unable to use complex interfaces.

Lastly, AI models should be able to sustain performance. The alteration of the surgery, rehabilitation regimen and demographics of the patients may worsen the accuracy unless retraining and monitoring of the patients are done continuously. Such limitations are important to be addressed in order to reliably use AI to provide predictive results of open tibial fracture.

4.12. Ethical, legal and regulatory considerations

The integration of AI predictive models with orthopedic trauma creates ethical, legal and regulatory issues that should be addressed in order to use them safely and responsibly. Privacy and data security is strongly prioritized in terms of protecting the privacy of patients and their data; this is more important given the vast clinical and patient-reported datasets that AI depends on. Trust and confidentiality can only be ensured through strong governance and adherence to data-protection regulations.

Clinical responsibility and accountability may also be considered as ethical factors. The use of AI predictions should be that of decision-supporting tools rather than supplants of clinician judgment. Strict separation of responsibilities will make certain that clinicians are held responsible in terms of making treatment decisions based on AI results. Excessive dependence on computer-generated forecasting without self-regulation may put the lives of patients at risk.

Explainability and transparency are related to ethical deployment. Patients and clinicians, at least, should have a conceptual understanding of how predictions are made and what factors motivate outcomes. Explainable AI methods assist in making improvements to the prediction to render it interpretable, justifiable and consistent with clinical reasoning keenly (Jasen 2025).

Regulative, AI clinical tools are under more and more regulation. The implementation of model validation, continuous monitoring of performance and post-deployment surveillance are a priority because authorities need to ensure the safety of usage and effectiveness. In particular, ongoing review is critical in the field of trauma care when the environment and guidelines evolve quickly.

Informed consent gains more importance. With the predictions of AI affecting rehab planning and return-to-work advice, patients must be informed about the use of AI in their treatment and the limitations to the predictions. It will be imperative to tackle these ethical, legal and regulating concerns using interdisciplinary teamwork to be able to integrate AI in orthopedic trauma practices in a responsible manner (Mennella et al. 2024).

4.13. Conclusion

AI-based models are an important step to predicting functional outcomes following open tibial fracture. These models are more accurate than the conventional methods because they combine clinical, surgical, rehabilitation and patient-reported data. Focus on functional recovery, rehabilitation pathways and projections about returning to work through AI are congruent with patient outcomes and aligned to their objectives of patient care. On the one hand, work continues on issues of quality, interpretability and ethics of data, but these issues should be tackled as more extensive clinical use grows due to ongoing technological and regulatory improvements.

The next step of the current research should be multicenter validation, explainable AI methods and seamless clinical integration to see AI as a chance to maximize treatment results in open tibia fracture patients.

4.14. References

Agarwal, S., Bhardwaj, C., Gatkamani, G., Gururaj, R., Darapaneni, N., Paduri, A.R. (2023). AI based employee attrition prediction tool. In *International Conference on Multi-disciplinary Trends in Artificial Intelligence*, 24 June, 580–588. Springer, Cham.

Beaulieu-Jones, B.K., Yuan, W., Brat, G.A., Beam, A.L., Weber, G., Ruffin, M., Kohane, I.S. (2021). Machine learning for patient risk stratification: Standing on, or looking over, the shoulders of clinicians? *NPJ Digital Medicine*, 4(1), 62.

Cirillo, E., Conte, C., Moccardi, A., Fonisto, M. (2025). Resilient AI in therapeutic rehabilitation: The integration of computer vision and deep learning for dynamic therapy adaptation. *Applied Sciences*, 15(12), 6800.

Cortez, A., Urva, M., Haonga, B., Donnelley, C.A., von Kaeppler, E.P., Roberts, H.J., Shearer, D.W., Morshed, S. (2022). Outcomes of intramedullary nailing and external fixation of open tibial fractures: Three to five-year follow-up of a randomized clinical trial. *JBJS*, 104(21), 1877–1885.

Cui, Y., 2024. An efficient approach to sports rehabilitation and outcome prediction using RNN-LSTM. *Mobile Networks and Applications*, 1–16. doi: 10.1007/s11036-024-02355-3.

Duong, H.P., Garcia, A., Hilfiker, R., Léger, B., Luthi, F. (2022). Systematic review of biopsychosocial prognostic factors for return to work after acute orthopedic trauma: A 2020 update. *Frontiers in Rehabilitation Sciences*, 2, 791351.

Fritz, B., Paul, H.Y., Kijowski, R., Fritz, J. (2023). Radiomics and deep learning for disease detection in musculoskeletal radiology: An overview of novel MRI-and CT-based approaches. *Investigative Radiology*, 58(1), 3–13.

Guo, L.L., Fries, J., Steinberg, E., Fleming, S.L., Morse, K., Aftandilian, C., Posada, J., Shah, N., Sung, L. (2024). A multi-center study on the adaptability of a shared foundation model for electronic health records. *NPJ Digital Medicine*, 7(1), 171.

Jasen, S. (2025). Explainable artificial intelligence in healthcare. In *Applied Artificial Intelligence in Business: Systems, Tools and Techniques*, Yaseen, S.G. (ed.). Springer, Cham, 615–624.

Kokkotis, C., Moustakidis, S., Giarmatzis, G., Giannakou, E., Makri, E., Sakellari, P., Tsiptsios, D., Karatzetzou, S., Christidi, F., Vadikolias, K. et al. (2022). Machine learning techniques for the prediction of functional outcomes in the rehabilitation of post-stroke patients: A scoping review. *BioMed*, 3(1), 1–20.

Kumar, A., Batta, P., Rathore, P.S., Ahuja, S. (2025). Secure healthcare data sharing and attack detection framework using radial basis neural network. *Scientific Reports*, 15(1), 15432.

Lokerman, R.D., van Rein, E.A., Waalwijk, J.F., van der Sluijs, R., Houwert, R.M., Lansink, K.W., Edwards, M.J., van Vliet, R., Verhagen, T.F., Diets-Veenendaal, N. et al. (2023). Accuracy of prehospital triage of adult patients with traumatic injuries following implementation of a trauma triage intervention. *JAMA Network Open*, 6(4), e236805.

Lorente, A., Pelaz, L., Palacios, P., Benlloch, M., de la Rubia Ortí, J.E., Barrios, C., Mariscal, G., Lorente, R. (2024). Predictive factors of functional outcomes and quality of life in patients with ankle fractures: A systematic review. *Journal of Clinical Medicine*, 13(5), 1188.

Marra, M. (2024). Data-mining innovative approaches in biomedical fields. Thesis, Università Politecnica delle Marche [Online]. Available at: https://hdl.handle.net/11566/329735.

Mennella, C., Maniscalco, U., De Pietro, G., Esposito, M. (2024). Ethical and regulatory challenges of AI technologies in healthcare: A narrative review. *Heliyon*, 10(4), e26297. doi: 10.1016/j.heliyon.2024.e26297.

Misir, A. and Yuce, A. (2025). AI in orthopedic research: A comprehensive review. *Journal of Orthopaedic Research: Official Publication of the Orthopaedic Research Society*, 43(8), 1508–1527. doi: 10.1002/jor.26109.

Nayar, S.K., Alcock, H.M., Edwards, D.S. (2022). Primary amputation versus limb salvage in upper limb major trauma: A systematic review. *European Journal of Orthopaedic Surgery & Traumatology*, 32(3), 395–403.

Nicolaides, M., Pafitanis, G., Vris, A. (2021). Open tibial fractures: An overview. *Journal of Clinical Orthopaedics and Trauma*, 20, 101483.

Ochen, Y., Peek, J., McTague, M.F., Weaver, M.J., van der Velde, D., Houwert, R.M., Heng, M. (2020). Long-term outcomes after open reduction and internal fixation of bicondylar tibial plateau fractures. *Injury*, 51(4), 1097–1102.

Peng, H.T., Siddiqui, M.M., Rhind, S.G., Zhang, J., da Luz, L.T., Beckett, A. (2023). Artificial intelligence and machine learning for hemorrhagic trauma care. *Military Medical Research*, 10(1), 6.

Saccomanno, M.F., Lädermann, A., Collin, P. (2024). Two-stage exchange arthroplasty for periprosthetic reverse shoulder arthroplasty infection provides comparable functional outcomes to primary reverse shoulder arthroplasty. *Journal of Clinical Medicine*, 13(3), 904.

Schade, A.T., Khatri, C., Nwankwo, H., Carlos, W., Harrison, W.J., Metcalfe, A.J. (2021). The economic burden of open tibia fractures: A systematic review. *Injury*, 52(6), 1251–1259.

Schurz, A.P., Wagemans, J., Bleakley, C., Kuppens, K., Vissers, D., Taeymans, J. (2023). Impairment-based assessments for patients with lateral ankle sprain: A systematic review of measurement properties. *Plos One*, 18(2), e0280388.

Shaikh, M.F., Yilmaz, E.B., Akinloye, O.M., Freitag-Wolf, S., Kachavarapu, S., Krekiehn, N., Glüer, C.C., Orwoll, E., Meyer, C. (2024). CNN-based osteoporotic vertebral fracture prediction and risk assessment on MrOS CT data: Impact of CNN model architecture. In *Annual Conference on Medical Image Understanding and Analysis*, 24 July, 42–57. Springer, Cham.

Shi, G., Liu, G., Gao, Q., Zhang, S., Wang, Q., Wu, L., He, P., Yu, Q. (2023). A random forest algorithm-based prediction model for moderate to severe acute postoperative pain after orthopedic surgery under general anesthesia. *BMC Anesthesiology*, 23(1), 361.

Tared, S., Khaouane, L., Hanini, S., Khaouane, A., Roubehie Fissa, M. (2024). Enhancing lung cancer prediction through crow search, artificial bee colony algorithms, and support vector machine. *International Journal of Information Technology*, 16(5), 2863–2873.

Tian, R., Zheng, F., Zhao, W., Zhang, Y., Yuan, J., Zhang, B., Li, L. (2020). Prevalence and influencing factors of nonunion in patients with tibial fracture: Systematic review and meta-analysis. *Journal of Orthopaedic Surgery and Research*, 15(1), 377.

Tian, C., Gao, Y., Rui, C., Qin, S., Shi, L., Rui, Y. (2024). Artificial intelligence in orthopaedic trauma. *EngMedicine*, 1(2), 100020.

You, D.Z. and Schneider, P.S. (2020). Surgical timing for open fractures: Middle of the night or the light of day, which fractures, what time? *OTA International*, 3(1), e067.

Zhang, Y., Zang, Y., Martin, R.L. (2025). Clinically most relevant psychometric properties of the Lower Extremity Functional Scale: A systematic review. *Disability and Rehabilitation*, 47(8), 1932–1938.

5

Implant Failure Risk Stratification in Orthopedic Trauma Through AI

Internal fixation, plates, screws and nails are common orthopedic implants used in the treatment of bone trauma to stabilize them and allow healing to take place. These implants have a relatively high failure rate, even with advances in materials, design, and surgical techniques, including the development of newer materials. Failures can lead to complications such as non-union, revision surgery, prolonged recovery, and increased healthcare costs. The causes of implant failure are numerous: patient characteristics, details of fractures, the forces that are exerted during the healing process and the decisions of surgeons. Conventional risk assessment methods are based on tradition and focus on limited variables; therefore, their accuracy and reproducibility are reduced. Machine-learning (ML) and deep-learning (DL) algorithms, which are part of artificial intelligence (AI), are the potential means of enhancing risk prediction. However, through integration of clinical, imaging and surgical data, AI models are able to identify nonlinear relationships that cannot be identified by traditional statistics. This review examines AI approaches for predicting orthopedic trauma implant failure, including data sources, algorithms, validation methods, current applications and limitations. It further discusses ethical, governance and implementation issues, as well as explaining recent developments and future opportunities. This chapter demonstrates the potential of AI to enhance clinical decision-making personalize trauma treatment and eventually decrease the number of implant-related complications.

5.1. Introduction

Orthopedic trauma poses significant global health challenges and contributes to long-term disability. High-energy fractures, including those caused by car accidents, industrial accidents, sporting activities and height fall are the most common sort of fractures. With urbanization, increased

Chapter written by Paresh PATIL and Dalavi Surekha GORAKH.

vehicle use, and an aging population, fracture rates are rising globally, placing a burden on the healthcare systems (Grønhaug n.d.). Most fractures are currently treated using inside–outside fixation devices: plates, screws, intramedullary nails and outside fixators. These types of devices help to recreate bone shape, provide mechanical strength and allow patients to move early, as this is essential for proper recovery.

Although implant technology, biomechanics and surgeon skill have improved, the issue of implant failure still exists as a clinical problem. Failure is where the fixation is unable to hold the bone stable until it heals, causing mechanical break-down, loss of alignment or poor healing. In the event of failure, patients would normally suffer delayed healing (Fan et al. 2021), non-union, misalignment, pain and poor functioning. They then require revision surgery, which is more complex, carries a higher risk of infection, is more time-consuming and most of the time results in suboptimal outcomes for the patient. Pre-emptive and accurate risk evaluation is thus important.

There are multiple causes of implant failure, which interact with one another. Bone healing is influenced by patient related factors such as advanced age, poor bone quality, cigarette smoking, metabolic disease, poor nutrition and other comorbidities. Fracture-related factors – including fracture type, location, severity, soft tissue damage, and fracture pattern – affect the mechanical environment. Surgical factors, including implant type, fixation method, quality of reduction, and postoperative weight-bearing, also play a critical role (Fan et al. 2021). The variables are interdependent with complex and, most times, nonlinear mechanisms, hence, failure is difficult to predict.

Historically, surgeons have been relying on their own experience, subjective cost and mere scores to determine failure. Although clinical expertise is essential, it is inherently limited, subject to bias, and may overlook incomplete or complex data. Classical statistical models, such as logistic regression, assume linear relationships and independent predictors, which do not adequately represent the complex biology and biomechanics of fracture healing. (Rupp et al.2024). Therefore, numerous at-risk patients could be overlooked during the preoperative phase, and others might be over-fixed.

In the recent past, AI has been a significant technology in healthcare that can enhance the accuracy of predictions and support clinical decision-making. ML and DL are part of AI and allow computers to discover the trends in vast datasets. In contrast to traditional models, AI algorithms are trained on the nonlinear interactions, which are complex, and improve with the increase in data (Cabitza et al. 2017).

Orthopedic trauma fits well with AI because the specialty generates much data. Electronic clinical records, X-rays, computed tomography (CT) scans, operative reports and follow-up notes form a deep digital trail, which can be modeled. By taking all these diverse sources and ensuring their integration into AI models, we can be guaranteed to receive personalized risk expectations, which is a less biased and more accurate evaluation of risk compared to regular techniques.

The clinical contribution of AI prognosis is big. With the right risk estimate in place preoperation, the kind of implant to use, the fixation approach and the surgical effort can also be precisely set. Surgeons can take care of every client based on their unique risk factors. Better fixation, biological add-ons or staged procedures may be beneficial to high-risk patients, whereas unwarranted complexity may be avoided in low-risk patients. During the postoperative period, AI-based monitoring can provide early warnings of construct failure, allowing timely intervention to prevent progression to severe complications.

AI is supposed to complement the surgeon's judgment rather than the substitution. As a decision-making aid, it will be able to provide care consistency, reduce variability and assist in evidence-based practice and keep the surgeon central to patient care. Successful adoption requires careful validation, transparency, and seamless integration into clinical workflows to ensure trust and usability.

With the growing adoption of AI in orthopedic surgery, it is timely to apply these technologies to the prediction of implant failure. This review summarizes existing evidence on the AI models for predicting fracture fixation failure, focusing on data sources, algorithms, clinical applications and barriers to implementation. By highlighting both its potential and limitations, this review aims to inform future research and support the responsible integration of AI into routine orthopedic trauma care.

5.2. Implant failure in orthopedic trauma: definitions and clinical significance

Implant failure is a key complication that undermines the goals of fracture fixation in orthopedic trauma. These goals include maintaining mechanical stability, restoring anatomical alignment, and enabling timely functional recovery. Implant failure generally refers to the inability of a fixation device to maintain stability until complete biological healing occurs. It may manifest in various forms, including mechanical breakage, bending or deformation, screw loosening or pullout, implant migration, and loss of reduction (Ghayyad et al., 2024). Clinical symptoms at the fracture site may include persistent pain, swelling, deformity, reduced range of motion, or functional deficits, often necessitating further interventions such as revision surgery or prolonged immobilization.

The rates of the implant failure are rather diverse and depend on a number of different factors: the nature and the place of fracture, the fixation technology applied, the bone quality and the comorbidities in a system. Mechanical complications are particularly likely to develop in high-energy fractures, comminuted fractures, periarticular fractures and osteoporotic bone fractures. Reported failure rates in multifaceted fractures range from approximately 5% to over 20%, indicating the significant clinical burden that this type of injury presents to clinics (Schömig et al. 2023). Implant failure not only worsens patient outcomes but also creates significant economic burdens, including prolonged hospitalization, increased healthcare costs, and a higher risk of medicolegal claims. (Ragland et al. 2020).

Biomechanically, implant failure occurs when mechanical forces exceed the strength of the fixation construct or bone. Key factors that increase mechanical load include inadequate fracture reduction, improper implant positioning or screw configuration, premature or excessive weight-bearing, and inappropriate selection of implant type or size. Although the best surgical method is applied, systemic and focal biological aspects can undermine bone healing and deteriorate mechanical instability. Osteoporosis, diabetes, smoking and impaired vascularity were recognized as factors contributing to mechanical instability (Roe 2020). In such a way, implant failure has a tendency to be due to the interaction of mechanical determinants with biological determinants.

Additional patient-specific factors influence the risk of implant failure. The bone–implant interface is weaker in older adults and in individuals with low bone mineral density. Comorbidities such as diabetes, rheumatoid arthritis, and chronic corticosteroid use further impair fracture healing. Lifestyle factors, including smoking and nutritional deficiencies, may delay bone union and contribute to early or late mechanical failure. Understanding these risk factors is essential for individualized patient management (Roe 2020).

To ensure the best clinical outcomes, correct risk assessment and timely identification of patients at high risk of implant failure are crucial. The traditional methods put much emphasis on the experience of the surgeon, subjective evaluation and independent clinical or radiographic parameters, which usually fail to capture the multifactorial relationship between the patient, fracture and implant variables. Different scoring systems and prognostic guidelines are suggested, although most of them are not highly sensitive and specific, particularly in complex or high-risk cases (Christensen et al. 2020). Therefore, there are a few cases where patients might not be discovered in time before they become complicated, and thus, they require revision surgery.

Since implant failure has clinical and economic consequences, more effective predictive strategies are desperately required. Risk stratification can be improved with the help of advanced computational tools, including AI, which can be used to evaluate multidimensional data, which encompasses patient demographics, comorbidities, fracture morphology, implant characteristics and postoperative aspects. The AI-based methods can provide better results, more objective and personalized evaluation, enabling surgeons to select the best fixation methods, modify the after-surgery procedures and take prophylactic measures (Christensen et al. 2020).

5.3. Rationale for AI in implant failure risk stratification

The nature of implant failure processes is complex, and failure is not easily predicted using conventional statistical and clinical instruments. Traditional regression models tend to postulate linear correlations among predictors and outcomes and preselect variables, restricting the scope of their ability to measure nonlinear relationships among variables, which fracture healing and implant biomechanics entail (Chen 2020).

AI offers the unique benefit that it can be used to recognize patterns through the interpretation of large and multidimensional datasets in an automated fashion. Clinical, radiological, surgical and biomechanical variables can be analyzed and used in parallel to predict risks in patients using ML algorithms to produce individual risk predictions (Lewandowski and Koller 2023). The models are type-adaptive since the amount of additional data keeps improving, and they can be used in dynamic clinical settings.

The other major advantage of AI-based risk stratification is personalization. In contrast to the averages at the population level, AI models provide patient-specific risk scores, which helps to choose implants and postoperative management plans individually (Dunka et al. 2021). Such an individualized method aligns with precision medicine, and it can reduce the under- and overtreatment.

Finally, the increased computing power and access to digital medical records and imaging repositories have spurred the use of AI in orthopedics. AI is not intended to replace clinical expertise; rather, its integration into clinical workflows can support and enhance surgical decision-making. Since orthopedic trauma care has a high cost of implant failure as one of the most common complications that may be avoided, AI-informed risk stratification is a promising option to enhance the overall outcomes.

5.4. Data sources for AI-based implant failure prediction

The quality, diversity and completeness of input data strongly determines the predictive performance of orthopedic trauma AI models. There is an intricate interaction between factors – patient-related, fracture-related, surgery and postoperative – that influence the risk of implant failure, and therefore, the combination of multidimensional data is crucial when determining the risk (Tian et al. 2024).

5.4.1. *Clinical and demographic data*

AI implant-failure models are based on clinical and demographic information. Key variables include age, sex, body mass index (BMI), comorbid conditions (diabetes, osteoporosis, rheumatoid arthritis), medication history (corticosteroid and bisphosphonate), smoking status and nutritional status. These factors are known to affect the healing of the bone and stability of the implants (Zand et al. 2022). The electronic health records, structural data (labs, prescription) and documented comorbidities can be turned directly into AI models, whereas the unstructured data (such as physician notes or surgical report) can be processed through natural-language-processing so that it extracts relevant clinical features. To predict risks at a person level, AI can include a wide spectrum of patient-specific information instead of basing the results on the average population levels.

5.4.2. *Radiographic and imaging data*

Assessment of fractures and fixation strategy is essential and is primarily achieved through imaging. Plain X-rays and CT scans and, occasionally, magnetic reasoning imaging (MRI) provide detailed data on the morphology of fractures, their displacement, comminution, bone density and involvement of the joints. After surgery imaging is used to analyze the position, alignment and mechanical disturbances of the implant. Convolutional neural networks (CNNs) are very effective in extracting subtle features of images without the manual process of image segmentation (Lindsey et al. 2018). They are able to see patterns that are associated with loosening, malediction or instability that might otherwise be unseen by clinicians to enhance prediction. Sequential imaging enables models to track the breakage healing process in order to detect the occurrence of mechanical defects at a nearby stage.

5.4.3. *Surgical and implant-related variables*

Intraoperative data have a critical impact on the mechanical stability of a fixation construct. The risk of failure is predicted by variables including type of implants, material, length, plate thickness, number and orientation of screws, as well as fixation geometry. Intraoperative precision, quality of fracture reduction and soft-tissue manipulation also have an impact on outcomes (Ajmera et al. 2021). The presence of this surgical information in AI models translates to a higher predictive ability due to the procedural variability and technical subtleties shared in AI-based models. The biomechanical parameters of load distribution, stress location and fatigue limits further refines the predictions of the model in an individualized setting.

5.4.4. *Longitudinal and postoperative data*

Dynamic postoperative data has the added value of predicting responses in relation to time with regard to fracture and fixation. Parameters such as progress in weight-bearing, adherence to rehab, serial imaging, bone-turnover indicators, as well as complications (infection, delayed union) may be inputted into AI models to streamline the risk estimates (Esteva et al. 2019). Longitudinal data can be best represented by recurrent neural networks (RNNs) and other time-series modes, which find the underlying temporal trends that provide indicators of the impending failure of the implant. Such data would transform the fixed preoperative instruments to dynamic tracking facilities to intervene before disaster failure.

5.4.5. *Data integration challenges*

Integration is a problem even though various data sources are promised. Heterogeneity in data, variation in image acquisition regimes, absence or incomplete observations and poor standardization have an adverse effect on model performance and extrapolation to different hospitals. Close care and annotation of the imaging and clinical data are also necessary to develop reliable models. The greatest potential for designing correct predictive systems is found in multimodal approaches that combine structured variables, unstructured text, image aspects and intraoperative factors. Table 5.1 provides the factors that lead to implant failure and data sources that are AI relevant.

Category	Specific factors	Examples mentioned in the paper	AI data source type
Patient-related factors	Demographics & biology	Age, sex, osteoporosis, diabetes, smoking, malnutrition, corticosteroid use	Electronic health records (structured data)
Fracture-related factors	Injury characteristics	Fracture location, comminution, displacement, soft-tissue injury, fracture pattern	Radiographs, CT scans
Implant-related factors	Hardware properties	Plate vs. nail, implant length, thickness, screw number and orientation	Operative records, implant databases
Surgical factors	Technical execution	Reduction quality, implant positioning, fixation geometry, alignment	Intraoperative notes, fluoroscopy images
Biomechanical factors	Load and stability	Stress concentration, construct stability, load sharing	Computational modeling, AI-derived features
Postoperative factors	Healing & rehabilitation	Weight-bearing protocol, compliance, delayed union, infection	Follow-up records, serial imaging
Longitudinal indicators	Temporal progression	Healing trajectory, early loosening signs	Time-series clinical and imaging data

Table 5.1. *Factors contributing to implant failure and their AI-relevant data sources*

5.5. ML and DL techniques

AI solutions to predict the probability of implant failure in orthopedic trauma can be broadly divided into ML and DL models. Each approach has strengths depending on the type of data, ranging from structured clinical variables to high-dimensional imaging data (Sasubilli and Kumar 2020).

5.5.1. *Supervised ML models*

Orthopedic outcome prediction shares features with supervised ML models. The labeled data that they learn are identified by the known outcome (implant failure). Common algorithms are logistic regression, support-vector machines, decision tree, random forests and gradient-boosting machine.

Logistic regression is easy and understandable but cannot deal with the multidimensional interactions in a complicated nonlinear fashion. These nonlinear relationships can be effectively modeled using support vector machines (SVMs) and ensemble techniques such as random forests and gradient boosting, which are well suited for processing high-dimensional data (Sahebhonar et al. 2022). Ensembles are used to group two or more learners to enhance robustness, alleviate overfitting and enhance accuracy.

The most important elements of supervised ML are feature selection and importance analysis. They determine which variables have the greatest impact on implant failure such as age, bone mineral, fracture type, reduction quality and the geometry of implants. This information is not only more accurate but also can provide clinically significant surgical planning information (Lauritsen et al. 2020). Supervised ML is the simplest way to unify heterogeneous data, such as clinical records, notes and biomechanical parameters, in one extensive prediction model.

5.5.2. *DL approaches*

Image-based prediction in orthopedic trauma had been redesigned with DL and particularly with CNNs. CNNs train themselves on hierarchical features in an automatic manner, discovering finer details that can be used to detect fracture complexity, the position of implants or the premature construct failure (Kong et al. 2022). In contrast to conventional ML, CNNs do not require feature engineering manually; thus, they are well suited to very large radiographic databases that cannot be annotated manually.

DL models are practical requirements. They need huge labeled datasets and large amounts of computer resources. In the case of few medical images, transfer learning, i.e. fine-tuning of already trained models, can be of use. Enhancing interpretability with attention mechanisms and saliency maps is becoming popular to allow clinicians to observe the parts of an image that cause risk estimates.

5.5.3. *Multimodal and hybrid models*

Combination models, which combine clinical structured variables with imaging-based features, have high potential. Multimodal neural networks can integrate demographics, comorbidities, laboratory results, surgical data, and imaging into a single model. These models capture both biological and mechanical determinants of failure and outperform single-modality approaches (Huang et al. 2020). Furthermore, RNNs and long short-term memory (LSTMs) are time-series DL structures that significantly improve prediction and yield a longitudinal postoperative data analysis, allowing healing to be monitored in real-time with instability identified promptly.

5.6. Performance metrics and model evaluation

Close inspection of AI models is crucial to ensure that they are trustworthy and have clinical significance in predicting implant failure. They should be evaluated not only for statistical accuracy but also for patient safety and the clinical relevance of the decisions they support (Camacho-Cogollo et al. 2022).

Such commonly used measures are accuracy, sensitivity, specificity and the area under the receiver operator curve (AUC). Sensitivity is essential in the studies of implant failures since failed positives may cause the delaying of preventive measures and disastrous failure (Deawjaroen et al. 2022). Specificity is also important to the extent that it avoids irrelevant invasive or expensive fixation strategies.

Calibration measures are used to test how closely predicted probabilities match actual failure rates, including the Brier score and the calibration plots. Well-calibrated models enhance clinician trust and support risk-based decision-making (Archer et al. 2022). Decision-curve analysis is a measure of the net clinical benefit at different risk levels (Wang et al. 2023).

Generalizability is checked by external validation using independent datasets. Early research frequently relied on single-center retrospective cohorts, limiting generalizability to other settings. More recent multicenter studies are more robust and highlight the importance of standardized reporting and clear validation procedures (Snell et al. 2023).

5.7. Clinical applications of AI-based risk stratification

Risk stratification based on AI can potentially revolutionize orthopedic trauma care, providing patient-specific predictions of implant-failures and assisting in preoperative evidence-based decision-making (Blake et al. n.d.). These are used for preoperative planning, intraoperative optimization, monitoring in the post-operative period and tailored rehabilitation.

5.7.1. *Preoperative decision-making support*

AI can be used to combine demographics of patients, comorbidities, bone density, fracture characteristics and previous surgery to identify individuals at risk of implant failure. Using this, surgeons will be able to design fixation plans and select the most appropriate implants. In high-risk patients, the methods that can be beneficial are dual plating, longer intramedullary nails or bone graft/biologic augmentation. Complex fixation is avoided in low-risk patients, to decrease the operation time, cost and complications (Maffulli et al. 2020). Preoperatively, AI also supports patient counseling and shared decision-making by providing objective risk estimates.

5.7.2. *Intraoperative optimization*

The introduction of AI into a surgical process provides real-time assistance. AI based on images is capable of evaluating the reduction, screw placement and alignment of the implants and screw positioning. Fluoroscopic image-analysis algorithms can detect inadequate reduction or implant placement and enable immediate intraoperative correction. Intraoperative decision support also reduces technical errors that may lead to mechanical failure, particularly in complex fractures or anatomically challenging cases. (Lauritsen et al. 2020). The load distribution and construct stability may also be predicted by AI, making appropriate adjustments based on the predictions prior to closing the surgical site.

5.7.3. *Postoperative monitoring and early intervention*

AI-based monitoring involves longitudinal tracking of patient progress. Temporal ML models can detect early signs of non-union, implant loosening, delayed healing, or abnormal stress patterns before clinical failure occurs. Early detection enables timely interventions, such as modifying weight-bearing, adjusting rehabilitation strategies, or performing preventive revision procedures, thereby reducing the risk of severe failure.

5.7.4. *Personalized follow-up and rehabilitation*

AI systems permit more targeted postoperative care by stratifying patients based on their predicted risk of failure. High risk patents may require more frequent imaging, increased vigilance and a more gradual weight-bearing protocol. Quickly rehabilitating patients with lower risk and limiting the number of imaging procedures are possible, which helps to maximize the available resources and ensure safety at the same time. This kind of personal approach enhances functional recovery and minimizes the number of visits to hospitals, cost of imaging and patient load (Rupp et al. 2024).

5.8. Ethical, regulatory and implementation challenges

Although AI has the potential to transform the stratification of implant-failure risk determination, there still are ethical, regulatory and practical issues. The major concerns relate to data privacy and security, which means that big data increases the concerns of ownership, consent and misuse (Roe 2020).

Another problem is algorithmic bias. In models trained on non-representative data, the performance of underrepresented demographics can be poor, as seen with the elderly, females or low-resource populations. Audits of fairness and various datasets are necessary to reduce bias.

From a regulatory perspective, AI decision support tools should meet medical device standards and undergo rigorous validation. The adaptive learning systems have no regular regulatory pathways, which is an obstacle (Deawjaroen et al. 2022). Black-box models are often distrusted by clinicians, and therefore, explainable AI techniques are increasingly necessary to ensure transparency and accountability.

Implementation challenges include integration with existing hospital information systems, potential workflow disruption, and the need for clinician training. Successful translation into practice requires an interdisciplinary approach involving surgeons, data scientists, and healthcare administrators.

5.9. Conclusion

The failure of implants is a multifactorial important issue in orthopedic trauma surgery, which negatively affects patient outcomes and becomes a burden to health care. Conventional risk appraisal based on clinical judgment and mere statistics is likely to fail to identify the intricate biological, mechanical and procedural interactions that culminate in fixation failure. AI is a highly dynamic solution to risk stratification, providing a data-driven response tool. Integrating clinical, radiographic, surgical and longitudinal data, AI models provide individual forecasts that can be used in pre-, intra- and post-operative planning and optimization. The promising results of AI in reducing implant-failure rates and decision support have been demonstrated by improvements in ML, DL and multimodal modeling, which demonstrate promising predictive accuracy. Nonetheless, there are issues of data quality, interpretability, bias, regulatory approval and clinical integration that have to be dealt with. With the ongoing development of research in the area with increased size of validation multicentric studies and the clarification of ethically sound AI, the incorporation of such technologies into daily orthopedic trauma practice is becoming more possible. Implant failure prediction based on AI is an essential step toward precision counter-cyclic orthopedic trauma treatment, leading to improved patient safety, utilization of the available resources and functional outcome quality in the long-term.

5.10. References

Ajmera, P., Kharat, A., Botchu, R., Gupta, H., Kulkarni, V. (2021). Real-world analysis of artificial intelligence in musculoskeletal trauma. *Journal of Clinical Orthopaedics and Trauma*, 22, 101573.

Archer, L., Koshiaris, C., Lay-Flurrie, S., Snell, K.I.E., Riley, R.D., Stevens, R., Banerjee, A., Usher-Smith, J.A., Clegg, A., Payne, R.A. et al. (2022). Development and external validation of a risk prediction model for falls in patients with an indication for antihypertensive treatment: retrospective cohort study. *BMJ*, 379, e070918. doi: 10.1136/bmj-2022-070918.

Blake, N., Kelly, D., Peña, S., Chanchal, A. and Chockler, H. (2024). Explainable AI for the classification of brain MRIs. *Research Square*. doi: 10.21203/rs.3.rs-4619245/v1.

Cabitza, F., Rasoini, R., Gensini, G.F. (2017). Unintended consequences of machine learning in medicine. *JAMA*, 318(6), 517–518.

Camacho-Cogollo, J.E., Bonet, I., Gil, B., Iadanza, E. (2022). Machine learning models for early prediction of sepsis on large healthcare datasets. *Electronics*, 11(9), 1507.

Chen, L. (2020). Overview of clinical prediction models. *Annals of Translational Medicine*, 8(4), 71.

Christensen, D.D., Klement, M.R., Moschetti, W.E., Fillingham, Y.A. (2020). Current evidence-based indications for modern noncemented total knee arthroplasty. *JAAOS – Journal of the American Academy of Orthopaedic Surgeons*, 28(20), 823–829.

Deawjaroen, K., Sillabutra, J., Poolsup, N., Stewart, D., Suksomboon, N. (2022). Clinical usefulness of prediction tools to identify adult hospitalized patients at risk of drug-related problems: A systematic review of clinical prediction models and risk assessment tools. *British Journal of Clinical Pharmacology*, 88(4), 1613–1629.

Dunka, V., Punukollu, P., Punukollu, M., Burugu, S., Yerneni, R.P., Kodali, S. (2021). AI-based biomechanical modeling for personalized orthopedic implants: Leveraging machine learning for patient-specific design, material selection, and post-surgical outcome prediction. *Essex Journal of AI Ethics and Responsible Innovation*, 1, 358–397.

Esteva, A., Robicquet, A., Ramsundar, B., Kuleshov, V., DePristo, M., Chou, K., Cui, C., Corrado, G., Thrun, S., Dean, J. (2019). A guide to deep learning in healthcare. *Nature Medicine*, 25(1), 24–29.

Fan, J., Xu, X., Zhou, F., Zhang, Z., Tian, Y., Ji, H., Guo, Y., Lv, Y., Yang, Z., Hou, G. (2021). Risk factors for implant failure of intertrochanteric fractures with lateral femoral wall fracture after intramedullary nail fixation. *Injury*, 52(11), 3397–3403.

Ghayyad, K., Escobar, P., Beaudoin, T.F., Wandersleben, L., Hawks, M., Ahmed, A., Kachooei, A.R. (2024). Nonunion fractures: Trends in epidemiology and treatment of femur fractures, 2017-2022. *Cureus*, 16(9), e70566. doi: 10.7759/cureus.70566.

Grønhaug, K.M.L. (2023). Intramedullary nails in the treatment of trochanteric and subtrochanteric fractures. PhD Thesis, University of Bergen, Bergen.

Huang, S.C., Pareek, A., Seyyedi, S., Banerjee, I., Lungren, M.P. (2020). Fusion of medical imaging and electronic health records using deep learning: A systematic review and implementation guidelines. *NPJ Digital Medicine*, 3(1), 136.

Kong, S.H., Lee, J.W., Bae, B.U., Sung, J.K., Jung, K.H., Kim, J.H., Shin, C.S. (2022). Development of a spine X-ray-based fracture prediction model using a deep learning algorithm. *Endocrinology and Metabolism*, 37(4), 674–683.

Kröner, P.T., Engels, M.M., Glicksberg, B.S., Johnson, K.W., Mzaik, O., van Hooft, J.E., Wallace, M.B., El-Serag, H.B., Krittanawong, C. (2021). Artificial intelligence in gastroenterology: A state-of-the-art review. *World Journal of Gastroenterology*, 27(40), 6794.

Lauritsen, S.M., Kristensen, M., Olsen, M.V., Larsen, M.S., Lauritsen, K.M., Jørgensen, M.J., Lange, J., Thiesson, B. (2020). Explainable artificial intelligence model to predict acute critical illness from electronic health records. *Nature Communications*, 11(1), 3852.

Lewandowski, N. and Koller, B. (2023). Transforming medical sciences with high-performance computing, high-performance data analytics and AI. *Technology and Health Care*, 31(4), 1505–1507.

Lindsey, R., Daluiski, A., Chopra, S., Lachapelle, A., Mozer, M., Sicular, S., Hanel, D., Gardner, M., Gupta, A., Hotchkiss, R. et al. (2018). Deep neural network improves fracture detection by clinicians. *Proceedings of the National Academy of Sciences*, 115(45), 11591–11596.

Maffulli, N., Rodriguez, H.C., Stone, I.W., Nam, A., Song, A., Gupta, M., Alvarado, R., Ramon, D., Gupta, A. (2020). Artificial intelligence and machine learning in orthopedic surgery: A systematic review protocol. *Journal of Orthopaedic Surgery and Research*, 15(1), 478.

Ragland, K., Reif, R., Karim, S., Sexton, K.W., Cherney, S.M., Stambough, J.B., Mears, S.C. (2020). Demographics, treatment, and cost of periprosthetic femur fractures: Fixation versus revision. *Geriatric Orthopaedic Surgery & Rehabilitation*, 11, 2151459320939550.

Roe, S. (2020). Biomechanics of fracture fixation. *Veterinary Clinics: Small Animal Practice*, 50(1), 1–5.

Rupp, M., Walter, N., Bärtl, S., Heyd, R., Hitzenbichler, F., Alt, V. (2024). Fracture-related infection – Epidemiology, etiology, diagnosis, prevention, and treatment. *Deutsches Ärzteblatt International*, 121(1), 17.

Sahebhonar, M., Gholampour, D.M., Kazemi, G.M., Soleiman, M.S. (2022). A comparison of three research methods: Logistic regression, decision tree, and random forest to reveal association of type 2 diabetes with risk factors and classify subjects in a military population. *Journal of Archives in Military Medicine*, 10(2), e118525. doi: 10.5812/jamm-118525.

Sasubilli, G. and Kumar, A. (2020). Machine learning and big data implementation on health care data. In *4th International Conference on Intelligent Computing and Control Systems (ICICCS)*, 13 May, 859–864. IEEE.

Schömig, F., Becker, L., Schönnagel, L., Völker, A., Disch, A.C., Schnake, K.J., Pumberger, M. (2023). Avoiding spinal implant failures in osteoporotic patients: A narrative review. *Global Spine Journal*, 13(1_suppl), 52S–58S.

Snell, K.I.E., Levis, B., Damen, J.A.A., Dhiman, P., Debray, T.P.A., Hooft, L., Reitsma, J.B., Moons, K.G.M., Collins, G.S., Riley, R.D. (2023). Transparent reporting of multivariable prediction models for individual prognosis or diagnosis: Checklist for systematic reviews and meta-analyses (TRIPOD-SRMA). *BMJ*, 381, e073538. doi: 10.1136/bmj-2022-073538.

Tian, C., Gao, Y., Rui, C., Qin, S., Shi, L., Rui, Y. (2024). Artificial intelligence in orthopaedic trauma. *EngMedicine*, 1(2), 100020.

Wang, W., Zeng, W., He, S., Shi, Y., Chen, X., Tu, L., Yang, B., Xu, J., Yin, X. (2023). A new model for predicting the occurrence of polycystic ovary syndrome: Based on data of tongue and pulse. *Digital Health*, 9, 20552076231160323.

Zand, A., Stokes, Z., Sharma, A., van Deen, W.K., Hommes, D. (2022). Artificial intelligence for inflammatory bowel diseases (IBD); accurately predicting adverse outcomes using machine learning. *Digestive Diseases and Sciences*, 67(10), 4874–4885.

6

Surgical Site Infection Risk Assessment in Orthopedic Procedures Using AI Tools

Surgical site infections (SSIs) are one of the major causes of postoperative complication in orthopedic surgery. They result in increased hospitalization, re-surgery, non-functionalities and increased expenditure on healthcare. Orthopedic surgery is particularly susceptible to infection due to the frequent usage of implants, sensitive nature of soft tissues and ability of bacteria to develop much-needed biofilms on prosthetic components. Although improved surgical methods and techniques, preoperative antibiotics and preventive measures have reduced the rate of infections, SSIs continue to occur due to the fact that the risk of infection, despite measures taken, is a complex issue and depends on the patient. Unconventional SSI risk methods are based on fixed scoring systems, linear statistical models and clinician judgment, and they do not always capture the intricate relationships between age, health history, surgical details and environmental conditions. Artificial intelligence (AI) is a potential solution to this because it offers superior and data-driven risk forecasts. With the use of machine-learning/deep-learning models, large and diverse datasets, such as electronic health records, lab findings, imaging and perioperative data, can be analyzed to generate customized, dynamic risk assessment. This review is a critical article on how AI tools can be used in the presence of SSI risk measurement in orthopedic surgery. It discusses the existing AI practices, data sources, model performance and clinical applications, and describes the issues of interpretability, data quality, ethics and real-world application. The review determines the capability of AI to detect high-risk individuals beforehand, facilitate preventive efforts and enhance the quality of surgery.

6.1. Overview of surgical site infections in orthopedic procedures

One of the most severe and problematic complications of orthopedic surgery is surgical site infection (SSI). This can lead to serious problems in the course of the postoperative stage, an increase in the length of

---

Chapter written by Jineshwar KAPALE and Attar Tabassum M.

hospitalization, dysfunction and increased healthcare expenditures. An SSI is an infection which occurrs at or near a surgical incision within 30 days of surgery, or up to a year afterwards if an implant is used. The application of prosthetic materials, which include joint replacement, plates, screws and spinal hardware, makes it difficult to manage infections, as they have the ability to absorb bacteria and develop biofilms. Such biofilms are unaffected by body defense mechanisms and antibiotics (Patel 2023). SSIs are a high-risk condition in the field of orthopedic surgery and warrant the primary attention of risk assessment, prevention measures and quality improvement.

Rates of SSIs differ significantly based on the orthopedic surgery procedure type, patients and hospital patterns. Elective procedures including primary total hip and knee replacement have lower rates of infection, between 0.5% and 2%. Complex surgery-revision arthroplasty, spinal instrumentation and fracture fixation have higher rates due to longer operating times, extensive tissue dissection and poor soft tissue coverage (Batty and Lanting 2020). There is also a high risk of SSI associated with trauma-related procedures, as they are usually associated with the urgent nature of intervention and the contamination of the sites of the injury, as well as a lack of the best pre-operative preparation of a patient (Edmiston and Leaper 2022). Although the percentages can be low, the actual number of orthopedic SSIs is high since the number of such procedures is growing across the world.

The effects of SSIs are far-reaching and multi-factorial. Patients require longer courses of antibiotics, repeated surgical clean-up procedures, removal or revision of implants and rehabilitation. The issue of prosthetic joint infections is particularly a problem; it can necessitate a complicated two-step revision operation, and these infections are associated with increased mortality, poor functional performance and poor quality of life (Natsuhara et al. 2019; Hartzler et al. 2020). In addition to personal consequences, SSIs have a significant financial cost of extending hospital stay, readmission and additional surgery and resource expenditure. Various reports indicate that the cost of a standard localized treatment of a prosthetic joint infection may be two to three times greater than that of a simple primary joint replacement, which poses the necessity of effective prevention (Natsuhara et al. 2019; Batty and Lanting 2020).

Staphylococcus aureus (including methicillin-resistant *Staphylococcus aureus* (MRSA)) and coagulase-negative staphylococci are the most common gram-positive causes of microbiologically determined SSIs in orthopedics (Kumar et al. 2025). There are also increasing rates of gram-negative and multi-drug-resistant organisms, particularly in trauma and revision cases. The interaction between pathogen virulence, biofilm formation and host immunity determines the development and severity of infection. The biofilms on the implant surfaces provide a protective response, where the antibiotics and immune system no longer work, thus necessitating surgery to eliminate the infection (Pérez-Laguna et al. 2021).

In orthopedic surgery, the prevention of SSIs insists on a multi-level strategy: prevention of surgical-related infections with antibiotic prophylaxis, optimal choice of operating methods, aseptic care and an individual approach to the mitigation of the risk. Despite this precaution, the rates of the infection are still high, as the traditional risk stratification instruments fail to embrace the complexity of risk of each patient. Although they are helpful, standard scoring systems and clinician judgment can be unsatisfactory at predicting which patients would be most susceptible to the development of SSIs when numerous coexisting risk factors are involved (Liu et al. 2024).

Emerging risk-assessment methods have a focus on information-based, customized tactics. Through the synthesis of electronic health records, the trends of labs, intraoperative information and characteristics of patients, a more detailed picture of SSI risk is created. The complex, nonlinear interactions of these variables can be predicted by advanced computational technologies, particularly AI and machine learning (ML), which provide personal estimates of risks that can be used to take specific preventive measures. Together, clinical knowledge and computational analytics will assist orthopedic teams in predicting high-risk patients, optimizing perioperative care and, finally, lowering the rates and effects of SSIs.

6.2. Risk factors for SSIs in orthopedic surgery

SSIs occur in orthopedic surgery as a result of a complex combination of patient-related, procedure-related and healthcare system factors. It is very important to know such determinants in prevention, risk assessment and personalization of care. Despite improved surgical performance and controls against infection, SSIs remain a persistent problem because SSIs flow from multiple and interactive causes.

6.2.1. *Patient-related risk factors*

Patient characteristics have a strong effect on SSI risk, as they affect immune response, tissue healing and bacterial colonization. Older people have an increased risk of a greater infection due to immunosenescence and a decreased capacity of the body to repair its tissues (Wang et al. 2023). Obesity is a significant risk factor; it is associated with reducing the perfusion of tissue, increasing wound tension and prolonging surgery due to delayed healing time, with a related increase in the chances of infection (Hasler et al. 2021).

Diabetes mellitus is a serious factor increasing SSI risk in orthopedic patients. Hyperglycemia inhibits neutrophils' chemotaxis and neutropenic granulocyte function, and interferes with collagen synthesis, which delays wound healing and promotes bacterial growth (Lai et al. 2022). Smoking causes decreased oxygenation and tissue repair, putting the person at even greater risk of infection (Jiang et al. 2020). Other patient factors – malnutrition, anemia, chronic renal failure and immunosuppressive therapy – also affect the ability to fight infections and repair damage (Maurer et al. 2020).

6.2.2. *Procedure-related risk factors*

Surgical characteristics are among the greatest risk factors for SSI. Longer operative times are always associated with higher rates of infection because of the prolonged exposure of tissue and opportunities for contamination (Yang et al. 2025). Procedure type is important, with elective primary arthroplasty having a low risk of SSI and revisions, and fracture fixation and spinal instrumentation having a high risk due to complexity, soft tissue compromise and implant use (Lee et al. 2023). Implants offer an attachment surface for bacteria and biofilm formation, which will complicate treatment and sometimes need additional surgery for removal (Lee et al. 2023).

Other intraoperative factors are loss of blood, treatment of tissue, asepsis and type of anesthesia. Proper timing and choice of prophylactic antibiotics also decrease the risk of infection (Wang et al. 2022). Emergency or trauma surgeries have a higher SSI risk compared to elective surgery due to a lack of optimization during the preoperative period, as well as the increased chance of contamination. Postoperative problems such as wound drainage, hematoma and early monitoring of the wound are also outcome-affecting problems (Yilmaz et al. 2024).

6.2.3. *Healthcare system-related risk factors*

Institutional and environmental factors are important in the development of SSI. Factors within the operating room environment such as ventilation, sterility, traffic and microbial exposure, along with high personnel movement, frequent door openings and inadequate sterilization, increase the risk of contamination. Surgeon experience and institutional volume are important, and high-volume centers and experienced teams tend to have reported lower rates of infection (Yilmaz et al. 2024). Variation in protocol adherence between institutions is one reason for differences in SSI outcomes.

6.2.4. *Interaction of risk factors*

SSIs are rarely due to a single factor; they arise from patient, procedural and system determinant interactions. For example, an elderly, obese diabetic patient for a long revision arthroplasty. Conventional models are usually unable to represent such nonlinear interactions, which limits the accuracy of the predictive models. AI-based models can pair the heterogeneous data and show complex relationships between risk factors (Wang et al. 2023).

6.2.5. *Implications for clinical practice*

It is the recognition of SSI being multifactorial that allows for a focused intervention. Preoperative optimization, i.e. glycemic control, nutrition and smoking cessation – a low start point risk – and intraoperative measures that have been shown to reduce the risk of SSI include operative time reduction, careful handling of operative tissue and selection of the implants, which are also employed. Institutional practices – diligent sterile procedures, environmental control of ORs (operating rooms), continuous quality improvement and quality control measure up to patient- and procedure-level measures.

6.3. Limitations of conventional SSI risk assessment models

The conventional orthopedic SSI risk models are based on conventional statistical methodology, standardized scoring and physician judgment. Although such techniques seem to enhance risk perception of infection and preventive strategies, they have high limitations that disrupt predictive capability and clinical utility. Most of the models apply logistic regression, which includes the assumption of linear and independent relationships among the predictors and the outcomes. The real-life scenario is that SSI formation is a multi-dimensional, nonlinear process that is stratified by multifaceted interactions among comorbidities of patients, surgical characteristics, microorganisms and health-system factors (Garrido Espeja and Couso 2020). These simplification assumptions restrict the range of the models in representing real-world situations.

Scoring systems are widely used since they are very straightforward and easy to work with, yet often contain only a small number of variables with constant weights, which limits their capacity to reflect patient-specific subtleties. As an example, healthcare providers may give two patients the same score, but the patients would differ drastically in terms of health profile, comorbidities and susceptibility to infections, but the model would categorize them as the same risk (Bustamante-Munguira et al. 2019). This is a failure of personalization, which will result in overtreatment or insufficient risk mitigation.

The other significant limitation is the low generalizability. Most of the models are constructed using single-institution, retrospective datasets or even limited groups of patients. Consequently, their application in other settings where the patients have other demographics, procedures or infection control measures usually degrades their performance (Gül and Akcay 2020). This creates a critical issue in the field of orthopedics, where there is a lot of variation in terms of procedures, implantations and the use of perioperative protocols.

The classical models are also non-dynamical. Once constructed, they are seldom modernized to suit changes in practice, surgical developments, microbial resistance or advances in perioperative therapy. In the long term, the result of this is model obsolescence and low reliability. Besides, the traditional methods primarily rely on the structured data, and much of the unstructured data such as the operative notes, imaging finding and clinical narratives, etc., are omitted and may provide important context to SSI risk.

Clinician risk assessment continues to play an imperative role, but may be varied, biased in thinking and limited in time, particularly in large-volume orthopedic departments of clinics. A combination of these restrictions emphasizes the necessity to apply adaptive, data-intensive solutions that will be capable of combining various information streams, take into account the multifaceted interactions and offer customized risk forecasts. This issue has prompted the increasing interest in the methods of SSI risk assessment related to orthopedic surgery based on AI. Table 6.1 shows the comparison of conventional and AI-based SSI risk assessment in orthopedic surgery.

Dimension	**Conventional SSI risk assessment**	**AI-based SSI risk assessment**
Core methodology	Logistic regression, risk scores, clinician judgment	Machine learning, deep learning, ensemble models
Data inputs	Limited clinical variables, fixed risk factors	Multimodal data (EHR, labs, imaging, operative data, notes)
Handling of risk factors	Linear, independent assumptions	Nonlinear modeling with complex interactions
Personalization	Population-based estimates	Individualized, patient-specific risk prediction
Temporal capability	Static, single-time assessment	Dynamic, longitudinal risk updating
Use of unstructured data	Rarely included	NLP of operative notes, wound images, radiographs
Predictive performance	Moderate discrimination, limited generalizability	Higher AUC, sensitivity and robustness across procedures
Clinical output	Binary or categorical risk	Probabilistic, graded risk stratification
Preventive decision support	Limited	Targeted prophylaxis, monitoring and intervention planning
Key limitations	Oversimplification, poor adaptability	Interpretability, data quality, ethical and regulatory concerns

Table 6.1. *Comparison of conventional and AI-based surgical site infection (SSI) risk assessment in orthopedic surgery*

6.4. AI and ML in healthcare

Artificial intelligence (AI) is a field that covers methods that simulate human intelligence such as reasoning, learning, pattern recognition and decision-making. In healthcare, AI has been quite transformative with explosive digital health data, enhanced computational power and novel algorithms. AI applications ranging from diagnostics, prognostics, treatment optimization, workflow management and clinical decision support especially match or exceed traditional methods (Lewandowski and Koller 2023).

ML, a subfield of AI, is the ability of the system to learn from historical data and make better predictions over time, without having any hand-written rules. Supervised learning algorithms (decision trees, random forests, support vector machines, gradient boosting) are very good at classification and predictions of risks. These methods take several predictors and nonlinearities into account, and are able to identify complex interactions. Unsupervised methods such as clustering, PCA (Principal Component Analysis) and dimensionality reduction help to find hidden patterns and phenotypes in patients. DL, which relies on multilayer neural networks, is good when we have high-dimensional data – for example, imaging, continuous signals and unstructured text (Rajkomar et al. 2019).

AI can be used to integrate different sources of data. Electronic health records containing lab results, imaging, genetics and clinical narratives put together whole risk models. This is particularly useful for SSIs, which are an interaction between patient health, procedural detail, environmental conditions and microbes. Unlike traditional regression, AI algorithms actually model these relationships in a dynamic way, which provides individual risk predictions.

Another strength is the constant learning. AI models are updated as new datasets arrive, keeping the models relevant with evolving surgical methodologies, treatment of infection cases and the variation of patient population. Real-time implementation provides real-time insights for clinicians for preoperative planning, intraoperative monitoring and postoperative planning, which will promote proactive interventions.

Despite its promise, the use of AI in healthcare is challenging. Interpretability is critical – predictions from many models, particularly deep learning networks, are often considered 'black boxes' that obscure the reasoning behind specific outcomes, leading to reduced trust and adoption. Model performance also depends on the quality and representativeness of data; biased datasets can result in inequitable or inaccurate predictions. Furthermore, ethical, legal and regulatory issues – such as patient privacy, data security and accountability – must be addressed to ensure safe and responsible deployment (Rajkomar et al. 2019; Lewandowski and Koller 2023).

6.5. AI-based models for SSI risk assessment in orthopedic procedures

AI models are an increasing way to predict SSI risk in orthopedic surgery and have much larger gains next to normal risk assessment tools. They work with large multi-dimensional datasets and try to find complex patterns among the patient demographics, procedural details and periprocedural variables. Some popular algorithms are random forests, gradient-boosting machines, support vector machines, neural networks and ensemble techniques. Each algorithm is good at dealing with nonlinearity, high dimensionality and missing data, respectively, which are applicable to various orthopedic cases (Wilson 2023).

Studies have shown that AI models are better than classic regression and scoring systems in predicting SSIs after joint arthroplasty, spine surgery and trauma procedures. By combining many sources of data, demographics, comorbidities, labs, surgery time, implant type, antibiotic prophylaxis, intra-operatives, etc., AI generates customized risk estimates to beat generalized scores (Hopkins et al. 2020). Ensemble models use different algorithms in combination to provide a consensus model, which can reduce the problem of overfitting, as well as improve the model's performance across patient groups.

DL breakthroughs have increased the predictive power of AI with the help of unstructured data. Convolutional neural networks are used to examine postoperative wound photos or X-rays for early signs of infection, and recurrent neural networks use temporal patterns in labs, vitals or med timings. Natural language processing (NLP) extracts useful information from operative notes, nursing reports and discharge summaries, adding further features that increase accuracy (Sarkar 2021). These tools can point out certain warning signs that may possibly slip from the attentive clinician, and this can then prompt care.

AI-based SSI predictions are tested using standard methods: area under the curve (AUC), sensitivity, specificity, precision and decision curve analysis. Many models have good discrimination with an AUC well above the logistic regression or scoring tools (Chang et al. 2020). Beyond single scores, potential risks are predicted by some AI models in a probabilistic manner, which means that clinicians may stratify the risk of patients into different risk categories and base treatment interventions on this risk, such as optimized glucose control, antibiotics or tightened postoperative monitoring.

There are still challenges associated with the implementation. Clinicians want to get precise explanations for the predictions made by AI, and "black" box models are often met with skepticism. Bringing AI into electronic health records and surgical workflows is crucial for real-time use. Continuous monitoring is needed to keep the model relevant, considering the evolution of the techniques and protocols. Still, SSI prediction with AI is a significant step towards the personalized prevention of infections and improved patient outcomes.

6.6. Data sources and feature engineering for AI-driven SSI prediction

High-quality data and good feature engineering are the keys to successful AI SSI models in orthopedics. The accuracy and generalizability of the models depend on a wide variety of complete and reliable inputs to the models. Electronic health records are the best source of rich data that provide longitudinal data on demographics, comorbidities, medication history, labs, vitals, operative data and postoperatives (Qiao et al. 2024). These structured fields make the combination of multiple risk factors and individual predictions possible.

Lab values are very important, as they represent immunity status, inflammation and metabolic control. Key markers are white cell count, C-reactive protein, erythrocyte sedimentation rate, hemoglobin and perioperative glucose. Intra-intraoperative variables – the length of surgery, blood loss, type of anesthesia used, type of implant chosen, whether antiseptics are given before surgery, the operating room conditions – provide much needed context. Operations such as drainage, wound appearance, early labs and postoperative complications such as hematoma increase predictive power (Chen and Baxter 2022).

Feature engineering is a process of giving raw clinical data in model-ready inputs for better performance. Normalization, temporal aggregation, trend analysis and interaction terms help algorithms to capture complicated relationships and dynamics. For example, increases in inflammatory markers may be a better predictor of SSI than absolute levels, and combining intra-operative details with patient comorbidities may reveal risk-amplifying interactions. NLP techniques are increasingly being used to mine useful information from the unstructured text that doctors, nurses and other healthcare professionals write – operative reports, nursing notes, discharge summaries, etc. Unstructured data can offer additional context that structured data may lack.

Imaging is another very important data source. Radiographs, magnetic resonance imaging (MRI) and wound pictures are all able to be run through deep learning, such as convolutional networks, to identify subtle signs of infection before being recognized by clinicians. Combining structured EHR data, unstructured text and imaging is the way to improve accuracy and generalization. However, there are challenges associated with multimodal integration including variable data quality, interoperability gaps, missingness and standardization needs between sites.

Data integrity and a measure against bias are critical for good AI. Imputing missing values, performing cross-validation and validating different populations help increase reliability. Choosing features based on clinical knowledge helps to ensure that models are based on genuinely predictive features. The AI-generating SSI prediction can be accurate and clinically meaningful using carefully focused data sources, data preprocessing and feature engineering that can be transferred across orthopedic practices.

6.7. Clinical integration, ethical issues and implementation issues

The transliteration of AI-based SSI risk assessment instruments into orthopedic practice demands clinical integration and other clinical and non-clinical considerations. For AI models to be functional, they should be well integrated into current electronic health record structures, be part of current clinical workflows and provide actionable predictions of risk at the time of occurrence. This integration allows doctors to use personalized SSI risk estimates to plan operations, make decisions during the surgery and manage post-surgical care, without potentially adding additional mental or administrative burden (Aung et al. 2021).

One of the important issues in clinical adoption is model interpretability. Many high-performing AI models, in particular, deep-learning networks, are what we may call a black box, and while they can make an accurate prediction, they are not very transparent in explaining how certain variables affect risk. Clinicians may be reluctant to assume the responsibility of the features of these opaque outputs, especially when high-stakes decisions are involved on whether to proceed to surgery, administer antibiotic prophylaxis or choose an implant. Explainable AI methods, such as feature importance rankings, visual decision aids and interpretable surrogate models, continue to be applied to increase transparency and develop clinician trust.

Ethics are extremely important when it comes to implementing AI in healthcare. Patient privacy and data security will have to be rigorously enforced, especially when large amounts of sensitive health information are used to build and deploy models. Robust evaluation, validation, bias evaluation and continuous performance monitoring of different populations are essential to ensure fairness and reliability (Ishengoma 2022).

Challenges in the law and regulation are also present. Accountability and liability come into play when clinical decisions are based on the output of an AI. Clear protocols for responsibility prevent the protection of the patient and clinician. Because the regulatory systems for AI are still in development, the use of acceptable guidelines for model validation processes along with safety and performance oversight post-deployment will be necessary to ensure the uniformity of efficacy.

Some of the implementation barriers are not limited to the technical and ethical issues. The effective adoption requires education and training of the clinicians so that they have an understanding of the model capabilities, limitations and appropriate use cases. A multidisciplinary partnership – data scientists, physicians, IT staff and hospital management – is a sure way to successful deployment. Integration must reduce clinical disruptions while increasing the clinical utility of the AI predictions.

Despite such difficulties, the information gathered by AI-based SSI risk assessment has huge potential for better orthopedic outcomes. AI risk prediction provides personalized and real-time guidance that can help to inform targeted preventive strategies, such as optimized antibiotic prophylaxis, enhanced monitoring of patients after surgery or optimized surgical planning. With excellent data governance, transparency, clinician engagement and adherence to ethics, AI systems have the potential to improve patient safety and help to reduce rates of adverse infection, as well as improve the use of resources in orthopedic surgery.

6.8. Conclusion

SSIs represent a major challenge for orthopedic surgery: complex, interacting patient, procedural and system factors are contributing to the problem. Traditional methods for risk assessment, while useful, can be difficult to use to grasp the multifactorial and nonlinear nature of SSI risk. AI tools provide a powerful alternative to gathering large volumes of heterogeneous data and generating individual and dynamically changing predictions. Current evidence indicates that AI models are superior to traditional approaches in many different orthopedic procedures. However, to bring biosignatures from the research phase to successful clinical translation, high-quality data, proper and thorough interpretation, ethical knowledge and easy workflow integration are necessary. With extensive validation, interdisciplinary collaboration and effective regulatory oversight, infection prevention and orthopedic surgical outcome improvement can be achieved through the application of AI-driven SSI risk assessment.

6.9. References

Aung, Y.Y., Wong, D.C., Ting, D.S. (2021). The promise of artificial intelligence: A review of the opportunities and challenges of artificial intelligence in healthcare. *British Medical Bulletin*, 139(1), 4–15.

Batty, L.M. and Lanting, B. (2020). Contemporary strategies to prevent infection in hip and knee arthroplasty. *Current Reviews in Musculoskeletal Medicine*, 13(4), 400–408.

Bustamante-Munguira, J., Herrera-Gómez, F., Ruiz-Álvarez, M., Hernández-Aceituno, A., Figuerola-Tejerina, A. (2019). A new surgical site infection risk score: Infection risk index in cardiac surgery. *Journal of Clinical Medicine*, 8(4), 480.

Chang, M., Canseco, J.A., Nicholson, K.J., Patel, N., Vaccaro, A.R. (2020). The role of machine learning in spine surgery: The future is now. *Frontiers in Surgery*, 7, 54.

Chen, J.S. and Baxter, S.L. (2022). Applications of natural language processing in ophthalmology: Present and future. *Frontiers in Medicine*, 9, 906554.

Edmiston Jr, C.E. and Leaper, D.J. (2022). Prevention of orthopedic prosthetic infections using evidence-based surgical site infection care bundles: A narrative review. *Surgical Infections*, 23(7), 645–655.

Garrido Espeja, A. and Couso, D. (2020). Introducing model-based instruction for SSI teaching in primary pre-service teacher education. In *Science Teacher Education for Responsible Citizenship: Towards a Pedagogy for Relevance Through Socioscientific Issues*, Evagorou, M., Nielsen, J.A., Dillon, J. (eds). Springer, Cham, 153–171.

Gül, M. and Akcay, H. (2020). Structuring a new socioscientific issues (SSI) based instruction model: Impacts on pre-service science teachers' (PSTs) critical thinking skills and dispositions. *International Journal of Research in Education and Science*, 6(1), 141–159. doi: 10.46328/ijres.v6i1.785.

Hartzler, M.A., Li, K., Geary, M.B., Odum, S.M., Springer, B.D. (2020). Complications in the treatment of prosthetic joint infection: When do they occur? *The Bone & Joint Journal*, 102(6 Supple A), 145–150.

Hasler, A., Unterfrauner, I., Olthof, M.G., Jans, P., Betz, M., Achermann, Y., Uçkay, I. (2021). Deep surgical site infections following double-dose perioperative antibiotic prophylaxis in adult obese orthopedic patients. *International Journal of Infectious Diseases*, 108, 537–542.

Hopkins, B.S., Mazmudar, A., Driscoll, C., Svet, M., Goergen, J., Kelsten, M., Shlobin, N.A., Kesavabhotla, K., Smith, Z.A., Dahdaleh, N.S. (2020). Using artificial intelligence (AI) to predict postoperative surgical site infection: A retrospective cohort of 4046 posterior spinal fusions. *Clinical Neurology and Neurosurgery*, 192, 105718.

Ishengoma, F.R. (2022). Artificial intelligence in digital health: Issues and dimensions of ethical concerns. *Innovation and Software*, 3(1), 81–108.

Jiang, C., Chen, Q., Xie, M. (2020). Smoking increases the risk of infectious diseases: A narrative review. *Tobacco Induced Diseases*, 18, 60.

Kumar, A., Batta, P., Rathore, P.S., Ahuja, S. (2025). Secure healthcare data sharing and attack detection framework using radial basis neural network. *Scientific Reports*, 15(1), 15432.

Lai, J., Li, Q., He, Y., Zou, S., Bai, X., Rastogi, S. (2022). Glycemic control regimens in the prevention of surgical site infections: A meta-analysis of randomized clinical trials. *Frontiers in Surgery*, 9, 855409.

Lee, C.R., Kim, C.W., Park, D.H., Kwon, Y.U., Yoon, J.M. (2023). Risk of infection after septic and aseptic revision total knee arthroplasty: A systematic review. *JBJS*, 105(20), 1630–1637.

Lewandowski, N. and Koller, B. (2023). Transforming medical sciences with high-performance computing, high-performance data analytics and AI. *Technology and Health Care*, 31(4), 1505–1507.

Liu, H., Wang, Y., Xing, H., Chang, Z., Pan, J. (2024). Risk factors for deep surgical site infections following orthopedic trauma surgery: A meta-analysis and systematic review. *Journal of Orthopaedic Surgery and Research*, 19(1), 811.

Maurer, E., Wallmeier, V., Reumann, M.K., Ehnert, S., Ihle, C., Schreiner, A.J., Flesch, I., Issack, P.S., Stollhof, L.E., Nüssler, A.K. (2020). Risk of malnutrition in orthopedic trauma patients with surgical site infections is associated with increased morbidity and mortality – a 3-year follow-up study. *Injury*, 51(10), 2219–2229.

Natsuhara, K.M., Shelton, T.J., Meehan, J.P., Lum, Z.C. (2019). Mortality during total hip periprosthetic joint infection. *The Journal of Arthroplasty*, 34(7), S337–S342.

Patel, R. (2023). Periprosthetic joint infection. *New England Journal of Medicine*, 388(3), 251–262.

Pérez-Laguna, V., García-Luque, I., Ballesta, S., Rezusta, A., Gilaberte, Y. (2021). Photodynamic therapy combined with antibiotics or antifungals against microorganisms that cause skin and soft tissue infections: A planktonic and biofilm approach to overcome resistances. *Pharmaceuticals*, 14(7), 603.

Qiao, S., Li, X., Olatosi, B., Young, S.D. (2024). Utilizing Big Data analytics and electronic health record data in HIV prevention, treatment, and care research: A literature review. *AIDS Care*, 36(5), 583–603.

Rajkomar, A., Dean, J., Kohane, I. (2019). Machine learning in medicine. *New England Journal of Medicine*, 380(14), 1347–1358.

Sarkar, A. (2021). Deep learning in medical imaging. In *Knowledge Modelling and Big Data Analytics in Healthcare: Advances and Applications*, Mehta, M., Passi, K., Chatterjee, I., Patel, R. (eds). CRC Press, Boca Raton, FL, 107–132.

Wang, H., Xiong, C., Yu, Z., Zhang, J., Huang, Y., Zhou, X. (2022). Research progress on antibacterial coatings for preventing implant-related infection in fractures: A literature review. *Coatings*, 12(12), 1921.

Wang, B., Wang, Q., Hamushan, M., Yu, J., Jiang, F., Li, M., Guo, G., Tang, J., Han, P., Shen, H. (2023). Trends in microbiological epidemiology of orthopedic infections: A large retrospective study from 2008 to 2021. *BMC Infectious Diseases*, 23(1), 567.

Wilson, A. (2023). CORR synthesis: Can decision tree learning advance orthopaedic surgery research? *Clinical Orthopaedics and Related Research®*, 481(12), 2337–2342.

Yang, Z., Wang, Y., Wang, Z., Li, J., Du, P., Meng, H., Zhao, K., Zhang, J., Li, M., Jin, Z. et al. (2025). Duration of surgical antibiotic prophylaxis and surgical site infection in orthopaedic surgery: A prospective cohort study. *International Journal of Surgery*, 111(1), 492–501.

Yilmaz, M.K., Celik, N., Tarabichi, S., Abbaszadeh, A., Parvizi, J. (2024). Evidence-based approach for prevention of surgical site infection. *Hip & Pelvis*, 36(3), 161.

7

Functional Recovery Analysis After Hip Fracture Surgery Supported by AI Analytics

Hip fractures are among the most severe injuries in the elderly, associated with prolonged hospital stays, functional decline, and increased mortality. Although surgical treatment – either fixation or arthroplasty – aims to restore mobility, postoperative recovery varies considerably between patients. This variation is based on a combination of factors, including age, sex, pre-fracture function, illnesses present, details of previous surgeries, amount of rehabilitation, mental health and the environment. Traditional statistical models along with intuition by clinicians often do not represent this complex and nonlinear process. In recent years, artificial intelligence (AI) methods, such as machine learning (ML) and deep learning (DL), have become very powerful in predicting outcomes, risk stratification, individual rehabilitation planning and continuous monitoring of progress. This chapter collates contemporary evidence on various applications of AI analytics to post-operative recovery of hip fracture surgery function. It evaluates the predictive models of gait, daily living activities, complications, mortality and discharge destination in addition to the digital health technology via AI, including wearables, mobile apps and remote monitoring. Key methodological issues, such as dataset quality, feature engineering, validation, explainability and bias reduction, are discussed within the clinical context. Ethical, regulatory and operational issues that impact the integration of AI into geriatric orthopedic care are highlighted. Overall, analysis of functional recovery aided by AI is promising to revolutionize rehabilitation management in hip fractures by enabling the identification of high-risk patients early, offering more efficient allocation of therapy and facilitating individualized recovery programs.

Chapter written by P.N. KULKARNI and Pisal Rutuja A.

7.1. Introduction

Hip fractures are one of the most severe injuries in the elderly globally and are strongly associated with the loss of independence, institutionalization and mortality (Verduijn et al. 2024). As populations age, the global incidence of hip fractures is projected to increase dramatically straining the orthopedic, rehabilitation and long-term care systems (Karayiannis et al. 2023). Even if surgery is done soon to stabilize the break and allow early movement, patients return to their previous level of function in a very variable fashion. Many survivors are still left with challenges of limited mobility, difficulty performing daily tasks, lower quality of life and an increased risk of disability in the future (Huette et al. 2020).

Recovery following hip fracture is dependent on many interrelated factors. These include age, sex, basic demographic information, clinical information about how many other illnesses a person has, how frail they are, muscle loss, nutrition, cognition and mood, specifics of the fracture, type of surgery, anesthesia, complications around the time of surgery and how much rehabilitation a person received (Skjødt et al. 2021). Social factors such as where someone lives and whether they have help from caregivers also play a factor. Because these elements are all changing and interacting with each other over time, it is difficult to predict recovery using simple statistical tools.

Standard prognostic tools typically assume linear models of correlation based on simple assumptions about input–outcome relationships in a regression model (Topol 2019). But hip fracture healing follows complex patterns that vary with time and are influenced by enormous amounts of information – from clinical notes, imaging, lab results, to measures of gait from sensors and symptoms from the patient. In this context, AI methods, in particular ML as well as DL, are a powerful alternative. These systems learn buried patterns from large heterogeneous data sets, improving predictions and automating the grading of risk and individual planning of rehabilitation (Senders et al. 2018).

Over the past decade, therefore, AI has been increasingly used in orthopedic research and practice. Initially, it was mainly used to identify fractures on X-rays; however, its scope has expanded to prognosis, prediction of complications, facilitating the clinical decision and digital tracking of recovery (Benedetto et al. 2022). In the area of hip fracture care, AI models have been used to predict mortality risk, risk of readmission, destination of discharge and risk of regaining function of the hip often better than traditional risk models (Diao et al. 2024). All of these advances fit in with the larger effort towards personalized precision rehabilitation medicine.

Although it is of great benefit to patients, integrating AI into the workplace of everyday clinical practice remains limited. Key hurdles are poor data quality, missing entries, lack of testing in other settings, algorithm bias, lack of transparency and lack of clear legal responsibility. For AI-supported recovery analysis to be of any real use, it has to complement and not replace expert judgment and team-based rehabilitation planning (Chen et al. 2022). Clinicians need clear and interpretable results that help facilitate shared decision-making and patient-focused goals.

This chapter presents the most current information regarding the analysis of functional recovery by AI following hip fracture surgery. It first covers the underlying methodology of AI in outcome prediction, then an overview of applications to prognostic modeling, digital monitoring and rehabilitaiton optimization. Implementation barriers, ethics and future research directions are also discussed. By bringing the evidence together from a number of different fields, the review wants to demonstrate how AI can responsibly enhance the depth of functional recovery assessment in geriatric orthopedic care.

7.2. Functional recovery after hip fracture: concepts and measurement

Functional recovery after hip fracture is a measure of how much mobility, independence in performing daily activities and total participation an individual returns to compared to the state before the fracture. Recovery takes place in a number of different areas – physical performance, cognitive functioning, emotional well-being, social reintegration. Because of this complexity, numerous evaluation instruments have been developed that measure various dimensions of function (Sun et al. 2024).

Performance-based measures are the most widely used method of measuring mobility. They include timed tests of walking, such as the Timed

Up and Go (TUG), measurements of gait speed and chair rise tests that assess the strength and balance of the lower limbs. These tests are objective, reproducible and can be used to predict falls, hospitalization and mortality. However, with the addition of pain, fear of falling and environmental factors, results may be affected, introducing variability into longitudinal data (Vaishnav and Desai 2025). In the immediate post-operative period, many patients are unable to do this type of tests, leading to missing data complicating outcome modeling.

Self-reported functional assessments are another important component of recovery assessment. Common instruments include Barthel Index, Katz Index of ADL, Lawton Instrumental ADL (IADL) scale and disease-specific questionnaires such as Oxford Hip Score. They get hold of the perceived independence of a patient and their difficulty with day-to-day activities. While these tools are informative in understanding the patient experience, their responses may be skewed due to errors in recall, cultural differences, cognitive impairment or when patients cannot respond themselves, they may use a proxy (Pu et al. 2025). As there is often a co-morbid with dementia or delirium, proxy data are often required, causing a change in the validity of the measurement.

A third approach has relied on global assessments of health and quality of life instruments: the EQ-5D, SF-12 and WHOQOL instruments. These tools summarize physical, psychological and social wellbeing but are not as sensitive to subtle changes in levels of mobility or ADL capability. Recovery is increasingly viewed as a journey rather than a discipleship. Longitudinal studies usually measure outcomes at discharge, 3 months, 6 months and 12 months after surgery. The greatest improvement is typically seen during the first 3–6 months, with a slower period of improvement; often some patients never fully regain previous level of function following a fracture (de Munter et al. 2022).

Recovery also depends on the access and severity of rehabilitation. Early mobilization, multi-disciplinary management of geriatrics and structured physiotherapy always prove outcome improving. Yet rehabilitation pathways are very diverse between institutions and countries, which adds to the heterogeneity of research data. Social support and living arrangements outline recovery – those who return to institutional care or have no caregivers typically report slower improvements in functioning (Alshami et al. 2025).

Functional recovery is not isolated and free of medical risk. Complications including delirium, pneumonia, venous thromboembolism and surgical-site infection can delay the need for rehab and permanently change outcomes. Comorbidities – cardiovascular disease, frailty, malnutrition and sarcopenia – also have a negative impact. Therefore, functional recovery occurs in the context of interacting biological, psychological, clinical and social systems. Traditional linear statistics will often overly simplify these relationships, making AI-based analytics appealing for its ability to model misunderstood complex and nonlinear interactions over time (Mahajan et al. 2020).

Standardization is also an important challenge. Studies have different definitions of recovery, and therefore comparing and doing meta-analyses is difficult. Moreover, outcome measures may not reflect things that are important to patients, such as living independently or returning to meaningful roles. As there is a growing use of outcome metrics by AI models, prudent choices of clinically relevant endpoints are important to prevent optimization of predictions that are not prioritized for patients (Li et al. 2021).

Continuous, remote evaluation technology is also emerging. These systems produce high-resolution data in the longitudinal domain and can move functional recovery analysis from episodic measurements obtained in the clinic into real-time digital phenotyping. However, it is difficult to derive clinically meaningful information from such data unless there are sophisticated AI algorithms to process noisy, high-volume and time series information – a natural synergy between digital health and AI analytics (Han et al. 2022).

Overall, the multidimensional and ever-evolving nature of functional recovery makes it a good candidate for analysis using AI. By taking performance metrics in conjunction with patient-reported outcomes, clinical variables and data from sensors, it is possible to construct a more intricate, nuanced view of recovery that is more representative of how patients experience the real world.

7.3. AI and ML in clinical outcome prediction

AI includes computational techniques that allow computers to acquire the ability to learn from data and make predictions or classifications based on the information without being explicitly programmed for this. In healthcare, the branch that has been applied most is ML, which models complex and nonlinear relations between predictors and outcomes. DL, a subset of ML based on neural networks with multiple hidden layers, is particularly suited to high-dimensional data such as images and continuous streams of sensor data (Dakhil et al. 2023).

In predicting outcomes after hip fracture surgery, supervised ML algorithms are most often used. These are linear logistic regression with regularization, decision trees, random forests, gradient boosting machines, support vector machines and neural networks. These models are trained on labeled sets of data in which the outcome, for example, independence in ADL at 6 months, is known. By analyzing patterns of manifestations in predictors like demographics, comorbidities indices, laboratory findings, peri-operative variables and rehab exposure, the algorithm determines the probability estimation of the outcome for the new patient (Volkov et al. 2023). DL models advance this instinct and take this one step further by automatically extracting latent features in the raw data (radiograph, gait signals or free text notes), eliminating the process of manually engineering features.

The key to ML success is access to massive and high-quality datasets with sufficiently represented classes of outcomes. In the context of care of hip fractures, there is frequently data from a hospital administrative system, national registries or prospective cohort studies. These sources offer a variety of different predictors, as well as some issues – missing data, inconsistencies in coding and selection bias. Techniques such as multiple imputation, synthetic minority oversampling and cross-validation help alleviate these limitations while lowering over-fitting. External validation on independent cohorts will still be important to ensuring models are generalizable outside of the derivation site (Liu and Zhang 2021).

AI-based models have demonstrated good performance in mortality, complications and discharge disposition prediction following hip fracture.

For example, the algorithms gradient boosting and random forest algorithms often perform better than traditional logistic algorithms for the prediction of mortality by capturing complex interactions between age, frailty and comorbidities burden and the peri-operative complexity. Some models have an area under the receiver-operating characteristic curve (AUC) values above 0.80 – thought to be a good discriminative ability in clinical prediction research (Nagappala et al. 2025). Likewise, ML models have been used to categorize patients who are likely to require institutional level of care after discharge, in order to aid in pre-emptive planning of rehabilitation resources and care arrangements with caregivers.

Beyond the global outcomes, AI has also been able to predict functional endpoints such as mobility status, likelihood to walk independently as well as recovery of ADL. Incorporating sensor-derived mobility metrics or detailed physiotherapy records in ML models has positive prognostic accuracy values compared with the conventional scoring systems. Natural language processing (NLP) techniques can be used to extract functional descriptors from free-text physiotherapy or nursing documentation, which will allow AI systems to make use of rich qualitative information that only recently has been underused for predictive analytics (Dakhil et al. 2023).

Explainability is very important in the field of clinical AI. Black-box models might be highly accurate, but have little insight as to why they were able to make that particular prediction, which could undermine clinician trust. To overcome this, techniques of explainable AI (XAI) such as SHAP (Shapley Additive Explanations), ranking of feature importance and partial dependence plots are being used more often. These tools are useful for identifying the relative importance of predicting factors that contribute to the risk estimate for the individual, which supports human–HAI collaboration and enables clinicians to validate that model reasoning is clinically plausible (Wang et al. 2023). Moreover, unintended biases may emerge in models identified through XAI – for example, if predictions are disproportionately influenced by factors such as age or institutional residence – prompting the need for recalibration or fairness adjustments.

AI prediction is also increasingly being used for pre-operative optimization and shared decision-making. Surgeons and geriatricians may be able to use risk scores generated by AI to counsel patients and families on expected recovery trajectories, probability of institutional care or the need for high-intensity post-official rehabilitation. In principle, such personalized prognostic information can be helpful for goal-concordant care as well as more efficient utilization of rehabilitation resources. However, reliance on AI without recognizing its uncertainties could lead to self-fulfilling prognoses – for example, withholding intensive rehabilitation from individuals deemed to be "poor recovery candidates". It is therefore critical for ethical deployment to have a balanced approach that considers AI as a decision support tool – and not an ultimate arbiter of recovery potential (Dawes et al. 2021).

Another emerging use is for continuous learning systems which update the prediction models based on new patient data over time. Such adaptive models are attractive where, in hip fracture care, treatment protocols, anesthesia techniques and rehab pathways are evolving over a period of time. However, adaptive AI needs strong governance to avoid drift in performance and make improvements to the model to prevent them from causing harm. Regulatory bodies are beginning to look at avenues for regulatory approval for ever-learning medical software; however, clear guidance is still emerging (Jakhar and Kaur 2020).

At the technical level, performance measures have to be interpreted carefully. Discrimination (AUC) does not in itself ensure clinical utility. Calibration (agreement between predicted and observed risks) is important too, particularly when predictions are used to guide threshold-based decisions such as referral to intensive rehabilitation or not. Decision-curve analysis offers insight into the net clinical benefit for a range of risk cut points and is increasingly recommended for the evaluation of AI. Transparent reporting including standards such as TRIPOD-AI and PROBAST-AI may help to even better enhance methodological rigor and reproducibility (Cha et al. 2023).

In summary, AI-enabled outcome prediction is an expansion of traditional prognostic modeling in the management of hip fracture that offers the ability to process high-dimensional, nonlinear data and merge different sources of information. AI systems can create more individualized and precise predictions of functional recovery. Their value, however, has to be ultimately predicated on the thoughtful clinical integration and interpretability and a sustained focus on fairness, transparency and validation issues.

The applications of AI in functional recovery after hip fracture surgery are given in Table 7.1.

Domain	AI techniques used	Input data sources	Predicted/assessed outcomes	Clinical utility
Prognostic outcome prediction	Logistic regression (regularized), random forest, gradient boosting, neural networks	Age, sex, comorbidities, frailty indices, lab values, surgical variables	Mortality, complications, discharge destination	Early risk stratification and counseling
Functional recovery prediction	Machine learning, deep learning	ADL scores, gait tests, rehabilitation records, sensor data	Walking independence, ADL recovery, mobility level	Personalized rehabilitation planning
Digital monitoring of recovery	Deep learning, time-series models	Wearables, accelerometers, smartphones	Gait speed, activity levels, fall risk	Continuous monitoring and early intervention
Rehabilitation optimization	Reinforcement learning, ML classifiers	Physiotherapy intensity, adherence, performance data	Optimal therapy intensity and duration	Adaptive, individualized rehabilitation
Natural language processing (NLP)	NLP, transformer models	Clinical notes, physiotherapy narratives	Functional descriptors, social determinants	Utilization of unstructured clinical data
Explainable AI (XAI)	SHAP, feature importance models	Outputs from ML/DL models	Predictor contribution to outcomes	Transparency, clinician trust
Ethical & fairness analysis	Bias detection algorithms	Demographic and socioeconomic variables	Model equity across subgroups	Fair and safe clinical implementation

Table 7.1. *Applications of AI in functional recovery after hip fracture surgery*

7.4. Digital health, wearable analytics and AI-supported monitoring of recovery

Wearable devices and digital health platforms have enhanced the prospect of monitoring functional recovery after hip fracture surgical procedure. Gait speed, stride variability, postural control, activity dose and risk of falling can be continuously recorded from accelerometers and gyroscopes, as well as pressure insoles, and smart walkers, and from smartphone movement sensors in everyday life. This type of continuous data makes sense for complementing clinic-based assessments – providing valid information with greater ecological validity as to how patients are really functioning in their homes and communities (Krogue et al. 2020). They also provide help in identifying mobility decline or functional stagnation at an early stage increasing the chances of identifying these in-between scheduled visit dates.

AI is critical to the conversion of raw sensor data into clinically viable information. Deep learning models are especially adept at picking up on temporal information in the high-frequency motion data, accurately detecting walking, standing, transfers and falls. These models can also identify subtle gait issues such as increased step-to-step variability or asymmetry that might lead to a delay of recovery or complications. AI-augmented tele-rehabilitation platforms analyze the performance of exercises performed by patients at home, provide automated feedback and alert the clinician when patients go beyond prescribed targets (Mu et al. 2021). Such devices enable rehabilitation intensity to be modified in real-time according to the functional ability of the patient rather than by episodic visits to the clinic.

The deployment of sensor–AI-based systems on a large scale raises methodological and ethical questions. Not every patient is comfortable with technology, and lack of cognitive processing ability, lack of technological savviness, frailty and socioeconomic barriers may result in limited uptake. Algorithmic bias can occur when models are being trained on data that under-represents certain demographic or clinical groups, and as a result, the models perform unevenly (Chen et al. 2023). Privacy is also a concern as there is constant monitoring that builds very personal digital footprints revealing daily routines and vulnerabilities in that individual's health. Robust governance, traditional consent and privacy respecting methods of learning such as federated or edge AI are crucial to responsible implementation.

Integrating AI metrics into geriatric orthopedic care calls for organizational change. Clinicians need to learn to interpret model outputs and triage alerts and use digital information in shared decision-making. Workflow redesign needs to be done to ensure that alert fatigue is avoided and AI recommendations are used to complement, rather than interfere with existing processes. Evidence-based guidelines on thresholds, escalation and documentation will assist in putting digital insights into action with a timely response. Importantly, AI-assisted monitoring should be patient-centered with an emphasis on empowering the individual, educating the individual, and co-design, as opposed to the notion of surveillance.

Despite these challenges, AI-enhanced digital health systems have great promises for analysis of functional recovery. They are capable of providing a bridge between being rehabbed in a hospital and continuing on into community life by providing a continuous picture of progress that is used to support proactive, adaptive care. As regulators and societies continue to recognize the role of AI in the clinical decision support, the use of digital recovery analytics in clinical practice in orthopedics and geriatrics will likely become part of the routine clinical workflow, provided that safety, transparency and equity are ensured (Shortliffe and Sepúlveda 2018).

7.5. Implementation challenges in AI-supported functional recovery analysis

AI analytics have great potential for prognosis and rehab planning post hip fracture surgery, and there are several major challenges to implementation in a real-world scenario. The first one concerns data quality and interoperability. Hospital information systems are often data-rich but inconsistent, as they store data in fragmented and incompatible formats, variable definitions, coding and temporal resolution. It is common to have missing data, especially with functional outcomes which are not always regularly collected. Rehabilitation data – data information – for example, physiotherapy sessions information or exercise adherence data – is often recorded as part of narrative text rather than structured data fields that need NLP capabilities for extraction. Without standardized datasets, AI models face the challenge of learning site-specific artifacts that lead to model generalizability challenges when means are generalized to new populations.

A second challenge is that of representativeness and fairness. Hip fracture largely affects frail older people, who might be under-represented in digital datasets because of cognitive impairment, a low level of use of technology or institutional residence. If the training data for AI models is composed mostly of healthier or more affluent patients, the model's predictions can be poor in marginalized or medically complex patient groups, maintaining the status quo. Fairness-aware modeling strategies such as bias auditing, subgroup performance reporting and re-weighting techniques are essential if equitable benefit is to be ensured.

Transparency and interpretability are also important obstacles in the acceptance of clinical applications. Clinicians need to know why a prediction was created in order to determine its plausibility and discuss it with patients and families. Black box algorithms which give scores of risks without explanation can create distrust and hinder shared decision making. Explainable AI tools help to fill this gap, but the explanations must themselves be clinically meaningful rather than mathematically based.

Workflow integration is also another practical concern. AI systems that depend on excessive data inputs or generate frequent alerts can inadvertently increase clinicians' workload instead of reducing it. Integrating these tools into electronic health record systems, along with providing intuitive visualizations and optimizing alert thresholds, can help minimize this burden and enhance usability. Equally important is the training and cultural adaptation of people in care teams, so that clinicians see AI as a tool they can use to support them, as opposed to it being a threat to their professional independence.

Finally, regulatory, ethical and legal structures for the AI-generating medical software are, nevertheless, in development. Questions exist in relation to liability when decisions based on AI information have a role in adverse outcomes, in ownership of data obtained and in secondary use of health information.

7.6. AI-enabled personalization of rehabilitation and care pathways

One of the most promising uses of AI is the personalization of the rehabilitation strategy. Traditional rehabilitation protocols tend to be standardized, the intensity and content of which are formed by clinician experience and service availability. However, recovery needs vary greatly from one patient to another. AI-derived risk stratification models can help identify people who are likely to benefit from increased or extended physiotherapy, early intervention with a geriatrician, nutritional support or psychological counseling.

Beyond static risk assessment, AI can support adaptive rehabilitation planning. For instance, information from digital monitoring platforms can show whether a patient's level of activity is lower than expected. Clinicians may then make adjustments to exercise goals, adjust pain management or make community therapy visits. Over the years, these forms feedback where actual functional data help realign intensity of care that aligns the treatment with the actual rather than assumed performance.

Multidisciplinary care conferences may also be served by AI-assisted dashboards synthesizing clinical, functional and social data on intuitive visualizations. These tools can include highlighting change over time, which will enhance the situational awareness of the team, and enable goal-setting in a team that includes patients and families. Importantly, human oversight still has a central role. AI should augment professional judgment instead of dictating decisions around care, especially where they require complex decisions that have a strong value dimension (e.g. discharge destination, transitions to long-term care).

7.7. Patient-centered perspectives and ethical considerations

Successful implementation of AI-supported recovery analysis needs to focus on patient values, preferences and autonomy. Many older people want to know their prognosis and may feel anxious when they are faced with probability estimates. Clinicians must therefore make sensitive predictions for patients based on AI, including describing the uncertainty in the results and the potential that they can be improved by rehabilitation effort.

Privacy and consent are important ethical issues particularly for technologies such as continuous monitoring technology that captures activity within the home. Transparent communication on what data is being collected and how it is being stored, along with who has access to it is essential. Patients should be able to withdraw from monitoring and not lose their ability to access care. Ethical deployment also includes making sure that there is accessibility for people with sensory impairment, low digital literacy or financial constraint to avoid the "digital divide".

Some scholars express concern about a phenomenon known as automation bias in which clinicians will excessively defer to algorithmic recommendations even when they are clinically counter-intuitive. Guarding against this requires training, organizational safeguards and the building of a culture Novas to learn and critically appraise AI rather than blindly accept it. At the same time, the principle of distributive justice should be taken into account, whereby it is necessary to ensure that AI-supported tools benefit the general population of hip fracture patients, and not a narrow group.

7.8. Future directions in AI-supported functional recovery analysis

Future studies would probably be conducted on multimodal data fusion with clinical data, imaging, wearable sensor signals, laboratory tests and patient-reported outcomes combined into unified prediction. The deep learning architectures that can process sequential and heterogeneous data may capture the recovery process better than single-source models. Federated and privacy-preserving learning strategies will allow for collaborative modeling across institutions using no centralization of data, over privacy and governance concerns while making datasets more diverse.

Another area of great promise is the creation of hybrid human and AI decision support systems that explicitly model clinical reasoning, in which the algorithmic predictions are crucial for decision support as well as use the probabilistic priors and rules based on clinical guidelines. Such systems may offer accuracy as well as transparency for enhanced clinician trust. Simulation-based AI could also be used for planning and forecasting services, including predicting resource needs for rehabilitation beds, home care visits and long-term care placement.

From a methodological perspective, there is a growing interest in strong external validation and the randomized evaluation of AI-supported care pathways and reporting standards that seem to be specific to rehabilitation research. Patient and caregiver involvement in the design of these AIs, using participatory and co-creation approaches, will help to ensure that the tools are used to address meaningful outcomes instead of more technical metrics.

In the longer term, AI-enabled recovery analytics may be a component in learning health systems, where the insights gained in routine practice can continually improve prediction models and individualization of care. Achieving this vision will require the strong interdisciplinary collaboration of clinicians, engineers, ethicists, policy makers and – importantly – patients and care givers.

7.9. Conclusion

AI has come up as a powerful tool that can analyze and make predictions about the functional recovery following hip fracture surgery. By combining high-dimensional clinical data, sensor-based data on mobility and patient-reported outcomes, AI systems are able to create unique risk profile, planning rehabilitation, covering continuous monitoring during the recovery process. These capabilities are actually promising for mobility outcome, independence in daily living and quality of life for older adults recovering from hip fracture. However, integrating AI into routine geriatric orthopedic practice must be done carefully to ensure the quality, transparency, fairness and ethical governance of data. AI should be used to aid rather than replace the clinical judgment of experts, and systems need to be thoroughly validated in a wide range of population groups before they can be widely deployed. Meaningful engagement of patients, effective communication of uncertainty and access to digital tools to support health literacy are key elements in ensuring that technological advances are translated into real world benefits. When applied responsibly in interdisciplinary care pathways, AI-supported functional recovery analysis can play a role in more personalized, proactive, patient-centered rehabilitation after hip fracture surgery.

7.10. References

Alshami, A., Nashwan, A., AlDardour, A., Qusini, A. (2025). Artificial Intelligence in rehabilitation: A narrative review on advancing patient care. *Rehabilitación*, 59(2), 100911.

Benedetto, U., Dimagli, A., Sinha, S., Cocomello, L., Gibbison, B., Caputo, M., Gaunt, T., Lyon, M., Holmes, C., Angelini, G.D. (2022). Machine learning improves mortality risk prediction after cardiac surgery: Systematic review and meta-analysis. *The Journal of Thoracic and Cardiovascular Surgery*, 163(6), 2075–2087.

Cha, Y., Kim, J.T., Kim, J.W., Seo, S.H., Lee, S.Y., Yoo, J.I. (2023). Effect of artificial intelligence or machine learning on prediction of hip fracture risk: Systematic review. *Journal of Bone Metabolism*, 30(3), 245.

Chen, P.F., Chen, L., Lin, Y.K., Li, G.H., Lai, F., Lu, C.W., Yang, C.Y., Chen, K.C., Lin, T.Y. (2022). Predicting postoperative mortality with deep neural networks and natural language processing: Model development and validation. *JMIR Medical Informatics*, 10(5), e38241.

Chen, R.J., Wang, J.J., Williamson, D.F., Chen, T.Y., Lipkova, J., Lu, M.Y., Sahai, S., Mahmood, F. (2023). Algorithmic fairness in artificial intelligence for medicine and healthcare. *Nature Biomedical Engineering*, 7(6), 719–742.

Dakhil, S., Saltvedt, I., Benth, J.Š., Thingstad, P., Watne, L.O., Bruun Wyller, T., Helbostad, J.L., Frihagen, F., Johnsen, L.G., Taraldsen, K. (2023). Longitudinal trajectories of functional recovery after hip fracture. *PLoS One*, 18(3), e0283551.

Dawes, A.J., Lin, A.Y., Varghese, C., Russell, M.M., Lin, A.Y. (2021). Mobile health technology for remote home monitoring after surgery: A meta-analysis. *British Journal of Surgery*, 108(11), 1304–1314.

Diao, X., Wang, X., Qin, J., Wu, Q., He, Z. and Fan, X. (2024). A review of the application of artificial intelligence in orthopedic diseases. *Computers, Materials & Continua*, 78(2), 2617–2665. doi: 10.32604/cmc.2024.047377.

Han, S., Zhang, R.F., Shi, L., Richie, R., Liu, H., Tseng, A., Quan, W., Ryan, N., Brent, D., Tsui, F.R. (2022). Classifying social determinants of health from unstructured electronic health records using deep learning-based natural language processing. *Journal of Biomedical Informatics*, 127, 103984.

Huette, P., Abou-Arab, O., Djebara, A.E., Terrasi, B., Beyls, C., Guinot, P.G., Havet, E., Dupont, H., Lorne, E., Ntouba, A. et al. (2020). Risk factors and mortality of patients undergoing hip fracture surgery: A one-year follow-up study. *Scientific Reports*, 10(1), 9607.

Jakhar, D. and Kaur, I. (2020). Artificial intelligence, machine learning and deep learning: Definitions and differences. *Clinical and Experimental Dermatology*, 45(1), 131–132.

Karayiannis, P.N., Warnock, M., Cassidy, R., Jones, K., Scott, C.E., Beverland, D. (2023). The painful truth of waiting for hip and knee arthroplasty in Northern Ireland: A cohort study of the worst NHS waiting lists for elective hip and knee arthroplasty. *The Bone & Joint Journal*, 105(7), 783–794.

Krogue, J.D., Cheng, K.V., Hwang, K.M., Toogood, P., Meinberg, E.G., Geiger, E.J., Zaid, M., McGill, K.C., Patel, R., Sohn, J.H. et al. (2020). Automatic hip fracture identification and functional subclassification with deep learning. *Radiology: Artificial Intelligence*, 2(2), e190023.

Li, Y., Chen, M., Lv, H., Yin, P., Zhang, L., Tang, P. (2021). A novel machine-learning algorithm for predicting mortality risk after hip fracture surgery. *Injury*, 52(6), 1487–1493.

Liu, Y. and Zhang, L. (2021). Federated learning for healthcare: Opportunities and challenges. *IEEE Journal of Biomedical and Health Informatics*, 25(11), 4153–4160.

Mahajan, S.M., Mahajan, A., Nguyen, C., Bui, J., Abbott, B.T., Osborne, T.F. (2020). Predictive models for identifying risk of readmission after index hospitalization for hip arthroplasty: A systematic review. *Journal of Orthopaedics*, 22, 73–85.

Mu, P., Dai, M., Ma, X. (2021). Application of artificial intelligence in rehabilitation assessment. *Journal of Physics: Conference Series*, 1802(3), 032057.

de Munter, L., van de Ree, C.L., van der Jagt, O.P., Gosens, T., Maas, H.A., de Jongh, M.A. (2022). Trajectories and prognostic factors for recovery after hip fracture: A longitudinal cohort study. *International Orthopaedics*, 46(12), 2913–2926.

Nagappala, S.B., Dhandi, S.S., McKegg, P.C., Driessche, A.M., Javid, K., Brennan, B., Pantuso, A., Ramappa, P., Hertzberg, M., Abbas, M., Hakeos, W. (2025). The impact of socioeconomic factors on the rate of discharge to rehabilitation following hip fracture surgery. *SSRN Preprint*. doi: 10.2139/ssrn.5404828.

Pu, H., Shu, X., Tan, F., Li, X., Qu, C., Peng, X. (2025). Machine learning for predicting extended length of stay in elderly patients with hip fractures: An enhanced recovery after surgery perspective. *Digital Health*, 20552076251406311.

Senders, J.T., Zaki, M.M., Karhade, A.V., Chang, B., Gormley, W.B., Broekman, M.L., Smith, T.R., Arnaout, O. (2018). An introduction and overview of machine learning in neurosurgical care. *Acta Neurochirurgica*, 160(1), 29–38.

Shortliffe, E.H. and Sepúlveda, M.J. (2018). Clinical decision support in the era of artificial intelligence. *JAMA*, 320(21), 2199–2200.

Skjødt, M.K., Möller, S., Hyldig, N., Clausen, A., Bliddal, M., Søndergaard, J., Abrahamsen, B., Rubin, K.H. (2021). Validation of the fracture risk evaluation model (FREM) in predicting major osteoporotic fractures and hip fractures using administrative health data. *Bone*, 147, 115934.

Sun, Y., Liu, Y., Zhu, Y., Luo, R., Luo, Y., Wang, S., Feng, Z. (2024). Risk prediction models of mortality after hip fracture surgery in older individuals: A systematic review. *Current Medical Research and Opinion*, 40(3), 523–535.

Topol, E.J. (2019). High-performance medicine: The convergence of human and artificial intelligence. *Nature Medicine*, 25(1), 44–56.

Vaishnav, A. and Desai, S. (2025). Revolutionizing stroke management with wearable technology: A narrative review of clinical applications, opportunities, challenges, and the future path towards equitable implementation. *Annals of Indian Academy of Neurology*, 10, 4103.

Verduijn, W.H., Sipers, W., Spaetgens, B. (2024). Optimizing orthogeriatric hip fracture care: Why fracture type matters. *Journal of the American Medical Directors Association*, 25(10), 105191.

Volkov, E.N. and Averkin, A.N. (2023). Explainable artificial intelligence in clinical decision support systems. In *IV International Conference on Neural Networks and Neurotechnologies (NeuroNT)*, 16 June, 3–6. IEEE.

Wang, J., Liang, Y., Cao, S., Cai, P., Fan, Y. (2023). Application of artificial intelligence in geriatric care: Bibliometric analysis. *Journal of Medical Internet Research*, 25, e46014.

8

Radiographic Evaluation of Bone Healing After Intramedullary Nailing with AI Support

Intramedullary nailing is the standard treatment for long bone fractures because of the provision of biomechanical stability, low invasion and the achievement of high union. Accurate evaluation of the healing process of the bone following intramedullary fixation aids in guiding the postoperative care and decisions surrounding weight bearing, as well as identifying the complication of healing such as delayed union or non-union. Conventional radiography remains the most common form of monitoring fracture healing, although it relies on subjective interpretations of callus formation, fracture gap reduction and cortical continuity. This relativity causes inter-/intra-variability and delays the required intervention. Artificial intelligence (AI), in particular machine learning and deep learning, now provides the possibility of an objective and quantitative analysis of radiographs. An AI system can automatically locate the fracture site, segment the callus tissue, quantify the healing progress and predict results for union from a series of images. These tools make the diagnosis more accurate, eliminate reliance on different observers and permit the detection of impaired healing in its early stages. Integrating AI into radiography evaluation can help to standardize fracture healing evaluation, increase clinical decision-making and promote personalized rehabilitation after intramedullary nailing. This review focuses on the biology of healing bones and radiography principles after intramedullary fixation as well as the shortcomings of traditional assessment and the rising role of AI technologies in the improvement of radiographic assessment and patient outcome.

8.1. Introduction

Fractures of long bones are a major component of musculoskeletal trauma and cause tremendous morbidity in all age groups. High-impact

Chapter written by Anupam S. KOLEKAR and More Seema NITIN.

injuries like those caused by road traffic accidents, industrial accidents, sports accidents and falls from a height often result in diaphyseal fractures of the femur, tibia and humerus. These are injuries that can create long-term functional impairment, loss of productivity and high healthcare costs. Effective surgical stabilization is necessary in order to restore alignment, obtain early mobilization and minimize complications associated with prolonged immobilization. Amongst the fixation methods available, intramedullary nailing is believed to be the gold standard of choice for long-bone shaft fractures due to the favorable biomechanical and biological properties (Bekos et al. 2021).

Intramedullary nailing has many advantages over other fixation techniques. It offers load-sharing mechanics, maintains the fracture hematoma, involves negligible soft tissue destruction and reduces the risk of infection. By positioning the implant within the medullary canal, along the mechanical axis of the bone, intramedullary nails are less vulnerable to the effect of axial loading and rotational forces and allow free controlled micro-motion at the fracture site. This environment promotes secondary fracture healing that is characterized by the accumulation of bone-forming callus and endochondral ossification (Wildemann et al. 2021).

Despite an overall high level of success rates, complications like delayed union, non-union, implant failure and malalignment continue to be important issues. These problems can make pain last longer, the recovery in function is delayed, more surgery is needed and there is an increased socioeconomic burden. Early recognition of impaired healing is therefore very important, to allow for intervention and better outcomes. Postoperative evaluation influences evaluation in weight bearing progression, the correct manner of rehabilitation and also the indication for further operations such as nail dynamization or bone grafting.

Radiographic evaluation is currently the mainstay for the follow-up of fracture healing after intramedullary nailing. Plain radiographs are very readily available, cost-effective and standard on follow-up (Atwan and Schemitsch 2020). These findings determine the amount of time in which the bone can accommodate an elevated mechanical load. However, radiographic interpretation is by nature qualitative and highly subjective based on the experience of clinicians.

One of the primary difficulties with radiographic assessment is the subjectivity of such an evaluation. Observers differ significantly with respect to their assessment of the callus size, density and cortical continuity, even with the experience of orthopedic surgeons and musculoskeletal radiographers. Variations in image quality, angles of projection and overlap of the implants make the interpretation even more difficult. Consequently, inter- and intra-observer variations remain and clinical decisions are inconsistent and inaccurate in determining true healing status.

Standardized scoring, such as the radiograph union score for tibia fractures (RUST), was introduced to help maintain consistency for the healing of fractures (Mısır et al. 2021). These systems do give a framework for structuring the evaluation, but they are semi-quantitative and rely on visual judgement. They describe radiographic appearance of the bone at a single point in time and do not recap the dynamic and continuous nature of bone healing. Moreover, they do not have high scores of predictive powers, and therefore their usefulness for predicting future healing outcome is low.

Another drawback of conventional radiography is that early biological healing is not visible. Cellular and molecular processes leading to fracture healing, such as inflammation, angiogenesis and osteogenic differentiation, take place well in advance of any structural adaptations that can be seen on radiographs. Therefore, biologically active fractures may not be visibly altered radiographically for several weeks and the roots of impaired healing may not be detected until late stages of healing (Kumar et al. 2026). This delay may delay clinical intervention and have a negative impact on outcomes.

In recent years, artificial intelligence (AI) has been making significant waves in the field of medical imaging, providing the ability to automatically analyze medical images, detect patterns and predict outcomes from these images. AI systems have reached the level where, particularly using deep-learning AI, the accuracy they can achieve is equivalent to, or better than, the accuracy of humans at certain tasks. In orthopedics, AI has been used in applications such as fracture detection, classification, implant evaluation and outcome prediction (Olczak et al. 2017).

The use of AI in the radiographic assessment of fracture healing is a logical consequence of these advancements. By analyzing large numbers of radiographs, AI algorithms are able to pick up subtle features of images and time patterns that might not be obvious to the human eye. AI-supported systems can offer objective, quantitative and reproducible assessments of the healing of the bones following intramedullary nailing, reducing dependence on observers and increasing diagnostic confidence (Prijs et al. 2022).

Furthermore, longitudinal monitoring of healing can be accomplished by serial analysis of radiographs driven by AI. Individual healing curves and predictions of likelihood for union or non-union can be created. These predictive insights could be used to support early clinical decision-making that helps to personalize rehabilitation strategies and prevent prolonged and/or failed healing.

This review focuses on the contribution of radiographical evaluation with AI to the evaluation of bone healing in cases of intramedullary nailing. It discusses the biological and mechanical principles of fracture repair, the limitations in conventional assessment of healing using imaging, emerging techniques for AI and their clinical implications. By combining innovations in AI with known orthopedic practice, radiographic evaluation of fracture healing may no longer need to rely on subjective interpretation but rather be applied using standardization, data-driven and patient-centered care.

8.2. Biological and mechanical principles of bone healing after intramedullary nailing

The bone healing that occurs after intramedullary nailing occurs predominantly due to secondary (indirect) fracture healing. This process involves inflammation, repair and remodeling and is controlled by biological and mechanical factors (Prijs et al. 2022). Unlike the absolute stability provided by rigid fixation, intramedullary nails provide relative stability. This permits controlled micromotion at the fracture site, which is essential for the formation of the callus and growth of the bone by endocrinal ossification.

The inflammatory phase begins immediately after the break. It involves the formation of a hematoma and the arrival of inflammatory cells and growth factors. These cells stimulate the growth of new blood vessels and cause the mesenchymal stem cells to become chondrocytes and osteoblasts

(Wu et al. 2024). Radiographs typically do not reveal any changes during this phase as the biological changes occur prior to visible changes in structure.

During the reparative phase, the soft and hard callus go through the two stages, respectively. The intramedullary nails allow the fracture to maintain its alignment while allowing axial macrostrain to occur. This macrostrain causes the callus size and strength to grow. The nail diameter, locking style (static vs dynamic), fracture location and pattern all have an impact on the mechanical environment and therefore the rate of healing (Bekos et al. 2021). Too high stiffness will prevent callus formation, and excessive stability will cause delayed healing or non-union.

The remodeling phase replaces woven bone by lamellar bone and restores the normal structure of bone. Radiographs of this reveal it as a slowly continuous cortex and a reduction in the callus size. Remodeling can then continue for a long time after the fracture appears to be healed, so conventional imaging does not always reveal the point where the healing is complete.

The understanding of the interaction between biology and biomechanics is necessary in order to interpret the X-ray findings following intramedullary nailing. Radiographic signs must be interpreted against the stability of the implant mechanically and biologically with respect to the patient.

AI-assisted radiographic analysis can be used to objectively quantify these healing patterns so that a correlation between the mechanical and biological outcomes can be made, allowing the prediction of the fracture union to be improved.

8.3. Conventional radiographic assessment of bone healing

Radiographic evaluation is the most common method for following healing following intramedullary nailing since it is available, inexpensive and is available for long-term follow-up. Standard anteroposterior and lateral plain X-rays are taken at regular visits to measure the progress of healing and the health of the implant (Schwarzenberg et al. 2020).

8.3.1. *Radiographic indicators of healing*

Important radiographic signs to look for are the evidence of callus formation, visibility of the fracture line, cortical bridging and alignment. Callus formation is the most visible sign of healing and is typically the first sign of healing and would be active biological repair. Increasing the callus size and density followed by cortical bridging across the fracture gap is a sign of progressing union (Atwan and Schemitsch 2020). The loss or obfuscation of the fracture line and reunion of the cortex is also indicative of successful healing.

However, the interpretation of these findings is subjective and may vary from observer to observer. Factors such as X-ray projection, picture quality and patient position will impact perceived healing. Intramedullary nails can cover some of the cortex, so it is more difficult to determine the quality of the bridging bone, particularly early on.

8.3.2. *Radiographic scoring systems*

To encourage more uniformity, scoring systems have been devised for tibial fractures, namely, the radiographic union score (RUST) and the modified RUST (must). These systems score each cortex individually, and points are awarded on the presence or absence of callus and visibility of the fracture line (Plumarom et al. 2021). Although these are better tools, which are more reliable than free-form assessment, they are still semi-qualitative and are based on visual judgments.

8.3.3. *Limitations of conventional assessment*

Plain X-rays offer only limited insight into callus composition, mechanical strength, and biological activity. The early stages of healing are often not visible, and delayed or impaired healing may take time to become apparent. Furthermore, classifying outcomes simply as union or non-union oversimplifies the inherently dynamic and continuous process of bone repair.

8.4. Limitations of traditional radiographic evaluation

Despite routine use, however, traditional X-ray assessment following intramedullary nailing has many inherent limitations that can impact upon clinical decisions. One of these main problems is the variability of the observer. Interpretation of the callus formation, cortical bridging and visibility of the fracture line is dependent on the experience of the physician performing the evaluation, which results in inconsistent evaluation among orthopedic surgeons and radiologists (Bizzoca et al. 2023).

Another limitation is that the visual manifestation of early biological healing is delayed. Cellular activity, new blood vessel growth and early matrix formation take place long before structural changes are seen on plain X-rays. Fractures which are biologically active but structurally immature may be mistaken for delayed union, and early symptoms of impaired healing may be overlooked until a later stage (Schwarzenberg et al. 2020).

Metal overlap impairs the clarity of the image and makes it more difficult to evaluate the cortical continuity of the brain, particularly when there is a lot of hardware in the way or the imaging angle is not optimal. Additionally, the study of radiographs only provides two-dimensional views of a three-dimensional biological process which limits the correct assessment of callus volume and distribution.

Radiographic scoring systems, although helpful for standardization, are of semi-quantitative nature and therefore unable to reflect the continuous and multifactorial nature of the bone healing process. These systems are also not predictive; they explain the current status but cannot make a good prediction of union or not union, for instance (Bowers and Anderson 2024).

Furthermore, recurrent radiographs result in cumulative increases in radiation exposure and healthcare costs, especially when there is a need for long follow-up with patients. These problems highlight the importance of advanced tools for imaging analysis providing objective, quantitative and predictive information.

AI-based radiographic analysis of this type of radiographic information addresses many of these difficult questions by automating image interpretation, reducing the dependence on the observer and allowing the early detection of abnormal healing patterns.

Table 8.1 shows a comparison of the conventional and AI-supported radiographic evaluation of bone healing after intramedullary nailing.

Assessment Aspect	Conventional Radiographic Evaluation	AI-Supported Radiographic Evaluation
Core principle	Visual interpretation by clinician	Automated, algorithm-driven image analysis
Key indicators assessed	Callus formation, fracture line visibility, cortical bridging	Quantitative callus area, density, symmetry, cortical continuity
Nature of assessment	Qualitative/semi-quantitative	Objective and fully quantitative
Observer dependency	High (inter- and intra-observer variability)	Minimal (standardized outputs)
Use of scoring systems	RUST/modified RUST	Automated scoring + continuous healing metrics
Temporal analysis	Single time-point comparison	Longitudinal healing trajectory modeling
Early detection of delayed union	Limited	Early identification via pattern recognition
Predictive capability	Descriptive only	Prediction of union vs non-union
Workflow efficiency	Time-consuming, manual	Rapid, automated processing
Clinical decision support	Indirect	Direct support for weight-bearing and intervention decisions

Table 8.1. *Comparison of conventional and AI-supported radiographic evaluation of bone healing after intramedullary nailing*

8.5. AI in orthopedic imaging

Medical imaging has seen AI become an extremely powerful tool in a very short period. It allows automatic interpretations of images, recognition of patterns and predictive analytics. AI systems imitate human mental functions and learn on big datasets and reveal convoluted associations in imaging data. In orthopedic imaging, AI has demonstrated great potential to increase the accuracy, efficiency and consistency of diagnosis (D'Angelo et al. 2022).

Machine learning (ML) is also a form of AI. ML algorithms take into consideration annotated data to give a prediction or classification. Conventional ML uses features, which are specified manually, for example, shape, texture and intensity. Deep learning (DL), and in particular, convolutional neural networks (CNNs), learn hierarchical features directly in the images. This renders DL particularly appropriate with respect to radiographic analysis (Yang et al. 2020). In plain radiographs, CNNs use bone conditions, fractures and injury localization better than other methods.

The use of AI in orthopedic trauma is not limited to detecting fractures. It is also able to examine the positions of implants, approximate bone age, screen for osteoporosis and anticipate postoperative results. Thousands of radiographs can be processed within minutes by AI to reduce the workload of clinicians and minimize diagnostic time. Reproducibility is also provided by these systems and variability in human interpretation is minimized (Srivastav et al. 2023).

The improvement in the imaging field has been due to enhanced computer capabilities, the use of vast volumes of annotated datasets and the improved quality of images. The application of AI in picture archiving and communication systems (PACS) is possible with embedded tools that facilitate the analysis of ordinary radiographs without interfering with existing procedures.

Successful implementation of AI requires quality training data and extensive validation on diverse populations and proper attention to ethics and regulations. AI is increasingly regarded as an adjunctive technology that enhances, rather than replaces, clinical judgment. However, challenges remain in achieving intuitive and reliable applications of AI in orthopedic imaging, particularly in assessing fracture healing after intramedullary nailing.

8.6. AI-based radiographic evaluation of bone healing

This problem attracts much attention because the assessment of bone healing after intramedullary nailing is objective and quantitative using AI. Serial radiography with the help of AI systems can identify possible patterns of healing that are not visible to the naked eye and enhance the accuracy and stability of the diagnosis procedure (Jin and Li 2024).

8.6.1. *Automated callus detection and quantification*

Another advantage of AI in the diagnosis of fracture healing is that the callus can be detected and segmented automatically. DL, particularly CNNs, identifies the fracture region, differentiates between the callus and normal bone, and measures the area, thickness, density and symmetry of the callus (Munasinghe et al. 2020). These measures allow comparison across the temporal dimension and between patients, reducing the subjectivity in the visual determination.

AI is also used to trace the course of healing, whether the callus development is comparable to the anticipated postoperative period. Early warning about abnormal patterns, for example, a less than adequate callus or asymmetry, causes quicker intervention.

8.6.2. *Prediction of fracture union and non-union*

Beyond descriptive analysis, AI models can predict the likelihood of fracture union or nonunion by integrating radiographic features with temporal clinical data. ML is trained on massive amounts of healed and non-heated fractures, and can discern subtle radiographic indicators of delayed or non-union (Takahashi et al. 2023). The predictive power helps to perform risk stratification early and to treat patients in a more personalized way.

Experiments indicate that AI prediction models are better than traditional scoring systems in predictive healing. Fractures at risk that are identified early before non-union will benefit from classic interventions, such as nail dynamization, biological augmentation or revision surgery that can potentially increase union rates and reduce morbidity (Chloros et al. 2021).

8.6.3. *Longitudinal monitoring and decision support*

AI actively analyzes radiographs sequentially and delivers healing curves and reports to clinicians. The longitudinal monitoring can support the data-driven decision-making and enhance communication with the patients regarding the progress. The AI will not substitute for clinical judgment; it simply supports the decision-making process.

8.7. AI models and algorithms used in bone healing assessment

The bone healing process is investigated using different AI models, where the majority of models are DL-based because of their more effective image processing and capacity to extract complicated spatial features based on radiographic input alone (Flynn et al. 2023).

8.7.1. *CNNs*

Most fracture-healing AI systems are based on CNNs. Architectures such as ResNet, DenseNet and EfficientNet extract hierarchical features and represent the morphology of the callus, cortical continuity and fracture gap features (Kshatri and Singh 2023). In ResNet, increasing network depth does not significantly hinder training due to residual learning, which improves the accuracy of interpreting complex images.

8.7.2. *Image segmentation models*

U-Net segmentation models, including variations, are typically resorted to in order to obtain accurate localization and measurement of the callus. They produce pixel-level labels defining the fracture locations, callus and cortical bone sites, which are important in quantitative analysis and long-term comparison.

8.7.3. *ML and hybrid approaches*

Radiographic features are also processed by traditional ML algorithms, such as support vector machines, random forests, gradient boosting, etc. Hybrid strategies are a combination of DL feature extraction and traditional classifiers to enhance their performance, particularly when using small datasets (Esteva et al. 2019).

Transfer learning reduces training time and enhances the prediction of generalized images by using previously trained models on massive spans of imaging data and fewer labeled radiographs as orthopedic targets.

The combination of these AI models offers a DL of bone healing, including the detection of features and the estimation of the outcome.

Redundant refinement and validation in different settings are needed in order to have reliable implementation, which would be clinically useful.

8.8. Integration of AI into clinical workflows

AI-based radiographic assessment should be incorporated into the current orthopedic environments to become clinically useful. The majority of fracture healing assessment AI systems are designed to run using standard PACS. They execute computerized analysis of regular radiographs with no interference with the existing imaging guidelines (Dikici et al. 2020).

Overall, after intramedullary nailing surgery, the automatic processing of postoperative radiographs is carried out using an AI algorithm. The system then locates the region of the fracture. Next, it measures and evaluates the growth of the callus, measures the bridging within the cortex and creates quantitative measures or healing scores. Such findings are presented in a format accessible to the clinicians. They may combine graphical healing curves, probability scores of fracture union or automatic indicators of delayed healing. This real-time decision support is more effective, and it reduces the mental burden on surgeons and radiologists.

There are also AI-assisted tools that standardize the follow-ups. They guarantee the consistent assessment by institutions and providers. This is particularly applicable in large-volume trauma centers in which numerous clinicians are involved with the same patient. AWP objective AI-based metrics are used in addition to clinical and patient-reported outcomes. They assist clinicians in choosing how to progressively increase weight bearing, dynamization of the implants or revision surgery (Lewandowski and Koller 2023).

The other benefit is enhanced communication with patients. AI systems create visual representations of the healing progression; these representations make patients cognizant of their recovery. When there is a better understanding, there will be an improvement in compliance with the rehabilitation procedures.

Implementation should be performed with training of clinicians, clear design of the algorithm as well as constant monitoring of the performance. Clinical judgment should not be substituted by AI systems, but rather it should be seen as a complementary tool that can supplement end-user clinical judgment. Considerate integration may greatly contribute to the management of fractures following intramedullary nailing.

8.9. Clinical impact and outcome improvement

The use of AI in the radiographic monitoring of bone healing in the presence of intramedullary nailing demonstrated a significant clinical effect. The systems that are AI-assisted enhance the quality of diagnostic results by offering objective and replicable evaluations of the progress of healing. They limit the variability exhibited by traditional visual interpretation (Novak et al. 2024).

The first consideration is that this will allow prompt diagnosis of delayed union and non-union. AI software is able to identify inconspicuous radiographic appearances and chronic healing designs that are not expected along their scale of progression. The early risk stratification enables clinicians to take action, such as nail dynamization, changes to weight-bearing protocols or bio-augmentation. These measures can avoid the development of non-union.

Personalized postoperative care is also made possible by AI-powered assessment. The quantitative healing measures allow the clinician to adjust rehabilitation and weight-bearing suggestions according to the healing rate of a patient. Such customized care can minimize complications due to premature loading but prevent the unnecessary immobilization of patients that exhibit a good healing process.

Systems, with the integration of AI, can help to optimize the use of resources. This minimizes unnecessary imaging, shortens the follow-up for simple cases and also minimizes revision surgeries. Efficiency and consistency with fracture measurements may also be useful in enhancing multicenter clinical trials through the standardization of radiographic endpoints.

One should keep in mind the fact that AI is not intended to displace clinical expertise. It should be used as a supplemental decision-support system. Integrating AI-generated knowledge into what is seen clinically, patient symptoms and functional findings results in more knowledgeable and resolute judgments. With the ongoing appearance of validation studies,

AI-assisted radiographic assessment tends to become an inseparable part of the contemporary orthopedic trauma treatment.

8.10. Challenges, limitations and ethical considerations

Although AI is potentially quite effective in assessing bone healing following intramedullary nailing, various issues have to be resolved to make the innovation more widespread. Data quality and variability is the major issue. AI algorithms require large outfitted datasets to train on. Radiographs, however, are different in terms of imaging protocols, exposure and patient positioning, as well as the types of implants used in different institutions. Such a heterogeneity may have an influence on model performance and generalizability.

The other limitation is whether the algorithm is transparent and interpretable. A lot of deep-learning models are black boxes, which do not give an apparent explanation of the mechanism to make decisions. Such non-transparency may decrease clinician credibility and medico-legal responsibility, particularly in cases where AI suggestions are contradictory to clinical judgment.

The problem of bias and equity is also important. Unless training data represents a variety of populations, AI models might not perform well in particular demographic groups or with different fracture patterns. There should be equitable performance based on age, bone qualities and comorbid conditions of deployment to ensure ethical deployment.

Regulative, AI-based medical imaging devices should be able to meet the changing safety, efficacy and data-protection guidelines. The privacy of patients and secure management of imaging records are important particularly when using cloud-based systems. There should be clear guidelines on the question of responsibility and liability in AI-assisted clinical decision-making.

Lastly, clinician education and adaptation of the workflow are needed to successfully implement AI. The unwillingness to embrace change, a lack of familiarity with AI tools and a perception of excessive dependence on automation might undermine the adoption. To find responsible solutions to these challenges, aspects such as transparent validation, user-centered design and constant observation play an important role in incorporating AI into orthopedic practice.

8.11. Future directions and research opportunities

AI technologies will be further developed and improved, and the result of using them in the assessment of bone healing after intramedullary nailing will be reported in the future.

Another possible direction is the creation of multimodal AI models that combine radiographic data with clinical variables, including age, comorbidity, fracture pattern, biomechanical stability and laboratory biomarkers. These integrated systems would be able to offer a more complete and individualized process of fracture healing.

Longitudinal and predictive modeling is another significant field of development. It is projected that in the future, AI systems will not just be based on a fixed image analysis but also on a dynamic analysis of serial radiographs, delivering customized healing plans and predicting the time to union with more accuracy. Such predictive conclusions could assist the clinician in streamlining schedules by arranging follow-ups and adjusting rehabilitation programs.

One research priority is to incorporate explainable AI (XAI) approaches. Increasing model interpretability through the use of convergent radiographic characteristics or regions that have effects on prediction will help in enhancing clinician trust and clinical adoption. Explainable outputs can also be used to train and educate orthopedic residents and junior clinicians.

The use of AI models should be validated in large, multicenter prospective studies that should involve a variety of populations and clinical settings. Using a standardized set of data and reporting frameworks will also be important in performance benchmarking and reproducibility.

Moreover, regulatory methods should be updated to be flexible to adapt to the adaptive AI systems that are enhanced as time goes by without jeopardizing patients.

With the ever-growing capabilities of computation and the influx of data, AI-assisted radiographic assessment could become an inseparable part of quality orthopedic treatment, benefiting patients undergoing intramedullary nailing.

8.12. Conclusion

Radiographic examination is still central to the observation of bone healing following marginal nailing, and the conventional evaluation procedures are constrained by subjectivity, inconsistency and lateness in detecting delayed recovery. AI can be an innovative idea in that it will provide an objective, quantitative and predictive way of analyzing the healing of fractures based on routine radiographs. AI-based systems improve diagnostic accuracy and limit the reliance of the observer, as well as the timely diagnosis of delayed union or non-union, which can support early and individualized clinical intervention. Although the issue of data quality, interpretability, ethics and regulation remain, ongoing technological innovations and validation testing are still enhancing the impact of AI in orthopedic imaging. AI integration into radiographic analysis is an important move towards data-wise, standard and patient-focused fracture management in the aftermath of intramedullary nailing.

8.13. References

Atwan, Y. and Schemitsch, E.H. (2020). Radiographic evaluations: Which are most effective to follow fracture healing? *Injury*, 51, S18–S22.

Bekos, A., Sioutis, S., Kostroglou, A., Saranteas, T., Mavrogenis, A.F. (2021). The history of intramedullary nailing. *International Orthopaedics*, 45(5), 1355–1361.

Bizzoca, D., Vicenti, G., Caiaffa, V., Abate, A., De Carolis, O., Carrozzo, M., Solarino, G., Moretti, B. (2023). Assessment of fracture healing in orthopaedic trauma. *Injury*, 54, S46–S52.

Bowers, K.M. and Anderson, D.E. (2024). Delayed union and nonunion: Current concepts, prevention, and correction: A review. *Bioengineering*, 11(6), 525.

Chloros, G.D., Kanakaris, N.K., Vun, J.S., Howard, A., Giannoudis, P.V. (2021). Scoring systems for early prediction of tibial fracture non-union: An update. *International Orthopaedics*, 45(8), 2081–2091.

D'Angelo, T., Caudo, D., Blandino, A., Albrecht, M.H., Vogl, T.J., Gruenewald, L.D., Gaeta, M., Yel, I., Koch, V., Martin, S.S. et al. (2022). Artificial intelligence, machine learning and deep learning in musculoskeletal imaging: Current applications. *Journal of Clinical Ultrasound*, 50(9), 1414–1431.

Dikici, E., Bigelow, M., Prevedello, L.M., White, R.D., Erdal, B.S. (2020). Integrating AI into radiology workflow: Levels of research, production, and feedback maturity. *Journal of Medical Imaging*, 7(1), 016502.

Esteva, A., Robicquet, A., Ramsundar, B., Kuleshov, V., DePristo, M., Chou, K., Cui, C., Corrado, G., Thrun, S., Dean, J. (2019). A guide to deep learning in healthcare. *Nature Medicine*, 25(1), 24–29.

Flynn, B.I., Javan, E.M., Lin, E., Trutner, Z., Koenig, K., Anighoro, K.O., Kun, E., Gupta, A., Singh, T., Jayakumar, P. et al. (2023). Deep learning based phenotyping of medical images improves power for gene discovery of complex disease. *NPJ Digital Medicine*, 6(1), 155.

Jin, M.L. and Li, M. (2024). Bone mineral density analyzed using artificial intelligence-based computed tomography: Association with fracture healing. *Journal of Medical Imaging and Radiation Sciences*, 55(3), 101578.

Kshatri, S.S. and Singh, D. (2023). Convolutional neural network in medical image analysis: A review. *Archives of Computational Methods in Engineering*, 30(4), 2793–2810.

Kumar, A., Batta, P., Ahuja, S., Rathore, P.S. (eds) (2026). *AI-driven Innovations in Physiotherapy and Oncology 1*. ISTE Ltd, London and Wiley, Hoboken, NJ.

Lewandowski, N. and Koller, B. (2023). Transforming medical sciences with high-performance computing, high-performance data analytics and AI. *Technology and Health Care*, 31(4), 1505–1507.

Mısır, A., Yıldız, K.İ., Kızkapan, T.B., Uzun, E., Özçamdallı, M., Oğuzkaya, S. (2021). Reliability of RUST and modified RUST scores for evaluation of union in pediatric and adult femoral shaft fractures. *Acta Orthopaedica et Traumatologica Turcica*, 55(2), 127.

Munasinghe, S.P., Somaratne, S., Weerakoon, S.R., Ranasinghe, C. (2020). Prediction of chemical composition for callus production in *Gyrinops walla* Gaetner through machine learning. *Information Processing in Agriculture*, 7(4), 511–522.

Novak, A., Hollowday, M., Morgado, A.T., Oke, J., Shelmerdine, S., Woznitza, N., Metcalfe, D., Costa, M.L., Wilson, S., Kiam, J.S. et al. (2024). Evaluating the impact of artificial intelligence-assisted image analysis on the diagnostic accuracy of front-line clinicians in detecting fractures on plain X-rays (FRACT-AI): Protocol for a prospective observational study. *BMJ Open*, 14(9), e086061.

Olczak, J., Fahlberg, N., Maki, A., Razavian, A.S., Jilert, A., Stark, A., Sköldenberg, O., Gordon, M. (2017). Artificial intelligence for analyzing orthopedic trauma radiographs: Deep learning algorithms – are they on par with humans for diagnosing fractures? *Acta Orthopaedica*, 88(6), 581–586.

Papachristou, D.J., Georgopoulos, S., Giannoudis, P.V., Panagiotopoulos, E. (2021). Insights into the cellular and molecular mechanisms that govern the fracture-healing process: A narrative review. *Journal of Clinical Medicine*, 10(16), 3554.

Plumarom, Y., Wilkinson, B.G., Willey, M.C., An, Q., Marsh, L., Karam, M.D. (2021). Sensitivity and specificity of modified RUST score using clinical and radiographic findings as a gold standard. *Bone & Joint Open*, 2(10), 796–805.

Prijs, J., Liao, Z., Ashkani-Esfahani, S., Olczak, J., Gordon, M., Jayakumar, P., Jutte, P.C., Jaarsma, R.L., IJpma, F.F., Doornberg, J.N. (2022). Artificial intelligence and computer vision in orthopaedic trauma: The why, how, and what. *The Bone & Joint Journal*, 104(8), 911–914.

Schwarzenberg, P., Darwiche, S., Yoon, R.S., Dailey, H.L. (2020). Imaging modalities to assess fracture healing. *Current Osteoporosis Reports*, 18(3), 169–179.

Srivastav, S., Chandrakar, R., Gupta, S., Babhulkar, V., Agrawal, S., Jaiswal, A., Prasad, R., Wanjari, M.B. (2023). ChatGPT in radiology: The advantages and limitations of artificial intelligence for medical imaging diagnosis. *Cureus*, 15(7), e41435. doi: 10.7759/cureus.41435.

Takahashi, S., Terai, H., Hoshino, M., Tsujio, T., Kato, M., Toyoda, H., Suzuki, A., Tamai, K., Yabu, A., Nakamura, H. (2023). Machine-learning-based approach for nonunion prediction following osteoporotic vertebral fractures. *European Spine Journal*, 32(11), 3788–3796.

Wildemann, B., Ignatius, A., Leung, F., Taitsman, L.A., Smith, R.M., Pesántez, R., Stoddart, M.J., Richards, R.G., Jupiter, J.B. (2021). Non-union bone fractures. *Nature Reviews Disease Primers*, 7(1), 57.

Wu, W., Zhao, Z., Wang, Y., Zhu, G., Tan, K., Liu, M., Li, L. (2024). Biomechanical effects of mechanical stress on cells involved in fracture healing. *Orthopaedic Surgery*, 16(4), 811–820.

Yang, S., Yin, B., Cao, W., Feng, C., Fan, G., He, S. (2020). Diagnostic accuracy of deep learning in orthopaedic fractures: A systematic review and meta-analysis. *Clinical Radiology*, 75(9), 713-e17.

9

Decision-Making in Polytrauma Management Enhanced by AI

The area of polytrauma management is one of the most challenging ones in terms of emergency and critical care medicine. It involves quick, precise and concerted decision-making in a variety of clinical fields. Complex patterns of injuries, physiological instability and incomplete information are characteristic features of polytrauma patients, putting severe cognitive and temporal pressure on clinicians. The old decision platforms, which include the trauma protocols and scoring systems, offer a structure, but they are usually incapable of responding in real time to changing patient conditions or processing large volumes of heterogeneous data. Artificial intelligence (AI) has recently become a new disruptive technology that can be used to improve clinical decision-making in polytrauma care. AI software processes multimodality data (prehospital setting, emergency rooms, images, operating rooms, etc.) by using machine learning (ML), deep learning (DL), natural language processing (NLP) and predictive analytics. They assist in diagnosis at early stages, stratification of risks, prioritization of triage, treatment planning and prediction of outcomes. This chapter critically analyses the use of AI to enhance the process of decision-making across the polytrauma spectrum, including the initial assessment and definitive care and recovery. It talks of the major applications, methodological developments, clinical deliveries and implementation issues. Ethical, legal and organizational factors are also addressed. Emerging trends include explainable AI, federated learning and real-time clinical decision-support systems. On the whole, this review highlights the possible benefit of AI for clinician expertise and enhancing efficiency, consistency and patient outcomes in polytrauma management.

9.1. Introduction

Polytrauma is the cause of significant mortality and long-term disability globally, particularly in young as well as economically productive groups. It

Chapter written by Vikas DESHMUKH and Piyush Ashokrao DALKE.

is characterized by the presence of more than one anatomical area or organ system with multiple traumatic injuries of which at least one is life-threatening when combined with the rest. These patients require timely, coordinated and precise decision-making prehospital, as well as in the emergency, surgical and critical care units. Morbidity and mortality can be significantly aggravated by any delays or errors.

The conventional methods are based on standardized procedures including ATLS (advanced trauma life support), clinical experience and trauma scoring systems. Even though these offer fundamental organization, they are frequently not able to represent the complexity and fluidity of polytrauma. Patients quite often report incomplete histories, have disturbed consciousness and quickly changing physiological parameters, making real-time decisions highly difficult. The increasing amount of data that comes with monitoring equipment, imaging, labs and electronic records can also be overwhelming for clinicians.

Artificial intelligence (AI) is proving to be of great value in decision-making improvement in a complex medical setting. AI systems, based on massive data, search for small patterns and produce predictions that a human being cannot discern. In trauma services, injury severity, prediction of mortality, optimizing triage, imaging and treatment planning are already using AI support (Yu et al. 2024).

Recent developments in ML and DL enable real-time, patient-driven decision-support technologies, which will constantly change depending on the patient's status. These technologies help to decrease the variability, enhance the diagnostic error and support clinicians to make timely and evidence-based decisions under pressure (Liu et al. 2025). With the transition of healthcare to precision and data-driven medicine, the idea of AI integration into polytrauma management is an essential step in trauma care.

This chapter will examine the role of AI in enhancing decision-making in polytrauma management. It discusses the existing uses, advantages and weaknesses, as well as suggests future studies and clinical aspects relying on the latest literature.

9.2. Decision-making challenges in polytrauma management

Polytrauma demands a complex decision-making approach because of unexpected injuries and time limitations. Patients are presented with several injuries, hemodynamic lability and altered mental status that hides the evaluation and makes care prioritization difficult. Clinicians need to rapidly detect life-threatening circumstances, select diagnostic courses of action and take time-sensitive interventions, often with poor information.

Information overload is one of the major issues. The current-day trauma care produces enormous amounts of data, including prehospital reports, continuous monitoring, laboratories, imaging and so on, as well as electronic records. Real-time synthesis of these non-homogeneous data streams can be very straining to metacognitive processes of group members and can also lead to poor and slower decision-making (Kang et al. 2021).

Clinician experience and availability of resources varies across institutions adding to variances. Although such protocols and scoring boundaries as the Injury Severity Score and Revised Trauma Score are useful, they cannot provide a picture of the dynamic evolution of injury and physiology (Lee et al. 2022). These instruments are not capable of continually adapting themselves to new information.

The other key issue is the problem of predicting patient courses: there is swift decompensation, massive transfusion is necessary, and the probability of complications such as sepsis or multi-organ failure is high. The proper process of prognostication is vital in the allocation of resources, surgical planning, as well as family counseling, which traditional methods fail to meet (Lee et al. 2023).

The issues of these are indicative of the constraints of the traditional frameworks and are indicative of sophisticated computing aids. AI is able to take multidimensional data and complex data and unearth patterns ignored, and it offers real-time predictions. AI can help reduce uncertainty, improve situational awareness and the quality of decision-making in polytrauma management by providing a data-driven suggestion (Ventura et al. 2024).

9.3. AI technologies in polytrauma care

The sphere of AI is very extensive and includes various ways of computing that are intended to replicate the processes of human learning, reasoning and recognition of patterns.

The use of AI in polytrauma care can be described as a tool that helps clinicians to transform complicated and diverse medical data into actionable information. In this environment, the most frequent AI products are ML, DL, NLP and reinforcement learning.

Numerous polytrauma decision support systems are based on ML. Supervised models are regular, for example, logistic regression, support washer machines, random forests and gradient-boosting trees and are used to classify risk and predict outcomes and estimate mortality (Baur et al. 2022). These models are based on the history of traumas and form a relationship between the variables of the treatment and patient outcomes and apply it to new patients.

DL has been particularly useful since it can handle data with extremely high dimension. Convolutional neural networks (CNNs) are particularly good at imaging, automatically detecting injuries such as intracranial bleeding, pneumothorax and damage on CT, among others (Peng et al. 2023). Time-series physiologic data are well addressed by recurrent neural networks (RNNs) and long-short-term-memory models to allow continuous monitoring of patients and predict deterioration early (Mayerhoffer and Ilić 2025).

The NLP system converts unstructured clinical documentation (e.g. emergency notes, radiology reports and operating summaries) into structured searchable information (Biswas et al. 2023). NLP will save time in documentation by converting narrative information into a format that may be combined with other variables and will enable real-time analysis.

Reinforcement learning is still in the emergent phase of clinical practice but has the potential to be useful in the individualization of treatment plans and resource allocation in rapid-moving trauma settings. Reinforcement models can propose adaptive interventions by studying the decisions made at any point in time to suggest effective interventions that can help to enhance the long-term outcome for patients (Hunter et al. 2023).

Combined, these AI methods provide a robust framework for improving decision-making across the polytrauma spectrum. When installed as part of daily processes, they facilitate ongoing educational experience, real-time analytics and personalized care, which enhances clinician knowledge and improves the quality of trauma care.

9.4. AI in prehospital polytrauma management

Pre-hospital attention is another variable that is dominant in determining outcomes among polytrauma patients. Quick identification, prompt response and the appropriate choice of transportation are a very important factor in survival and functional recovery. Decision-making is also challenging at the scene due to poor diagnostics and time constraints as well as field testing. The triage, risks evaluation and communication with receiving trauma centers are useful purposes of AI.

Vital signs, injury mechanism, demographics and environmental factors are examples of prehospital data used to create machine learning models with better predictive accuracy of severely injured patients compared to conventional triage rules (Toy et al. 2024). These triage assistants powered by AI help paramedics determine the severity of injuries and signal forward the patients requiring rapid admission to high-level traumas.

Smartwatches and smartphones that monitor the vital signs and vital organs provide AI with the opportunity to monitor several major parameters of physiologic parameters: heart rate, blood pressure, oxygen saturation and respiratory rate. Occult shock or degradation is identified early, and therefore, intervention is rapid, and a warning is implemented in advance to hospital teams (Rajaei et al. 2023). This preventative communication minimizes waiting time at the arrival of the patient.

Another layer is the use of geospatial and predictive analytics that can be used to optimize transport logistics. Using the degree of injuries, distance, traffic and hospital capacity, AI will be able to recommend the most appropriate destination trauma center (Choi et al. 2023). Evidence-perspective routing will reduce the transport time, and they will find themselves at facilities capable of handling complex polytrauma cases.

All in all, AI supplements situational awareness by inputting information-based knowledge into clinical reasoning. The adoption of AI in the emergency medical sector can reduce the rate of under- and over-triage, enhance the coordination between the prehospital and in-hospital units and eventually increase the success of polytrauma patients.

9.5. Emergency department triage and early assessment

The initial in-hospital touchpoint of polytrauma patients in the emergency department will be essential, where fast triage and precise evaluation will be crucial in preventing secondary injury to avoid deaths. However, most clinicians are faced with issues of overcrowding, time constraints and information overload, and this aspect undermines decision-making. It is a fast environment that is sharpened with the help of AI tools to enhance early assessment and triage.

Triage systems based on AI take in real USD data, including vital signs, lab, observation and so forth, to evaluate the acuity of the patient and their probability of decline. In the case of traditional scoring systems, ML has been superior in identifying those who are at risk of hemorrhagic shock, massive transfusion or even early death (Adebayo et al. 2023). The system receives new data, making predictions dynamic, which ensures that the patient status can be re-evaluated dynamically.

Continuous physiologic DL models of continuous data reveal insidious patterns of early shock or respiratory failure before obvious events (Xu et al. 2024). These alerts allow clinicians to intervene before the condition of the patient deteriorates and enhance outcomes and stabilization. In addition to this, AI decision support may be used to direct the selection of diagnostic studies and specialists to include and to utilize scarce resources optimally.

NLP is also used to reduce the burden as the task quickly retrieves useful information on the electronic records, ambulance data and previous histories. NLP minimizes the stress experienced by clinicians and allows them to focus on hands-on care by summarizing the main points and distinguishing risk factors (Zhang et al. 2024).

Finally, AI-assisted preliminary evaluation helps with information exchange between trauma groups. Intuitive knowledge disseminated between departments helps make unanimous decisions and reduce the variation in treatment. All in all, the introduction of AI into emergency department triage and assessment improves the triage and assessment of polytrauma patients.

9.6. AI-enhanced imaging and diagnostic decision-making

Making diagnoses and dealing with polytrauma involve imaging, and it is critical to identify life-threatening injuries in a short time to provide timely care. A CT of the whole body is now standard in severe trauma cases, but the increasing size and complexity of images can slow down the diagnosis and bring inconsistency into interpretation. AI has significantly enhanced the imaging-based decision-making process by accelerating, refining and standardizing the process of injury detection.

CNNs and other DL algorithms have been demonstrated to be accurate in detecting injuries such as intracranial hemorrhage, cervical spine, pneumothorax and solid-organ injuries on images (Li et al. 2025). These AI systems are able to quickly process a large quantity of images and mark dangerous results, which clinicians can review on the spot reducing the diagnosis period.

AI-assisted imaging tools also enable quantitative evaluation of injuries. Objective data that is provided through automated calculations of volume of hemorrhage, size of organ laceration and displacement of fracture is used to make a decision based on which treatment and surgical planning are made (Zia et al. 2022). Standardized measurements minimize inter-observer reliability as well as enhance inter-hospital reproducibility.

In addition to detection, AI models use image findings with clinical and laboratory analysis to predict such outcomes as surgery, intensive care unit (ICU) hospitalization or mortality (Swain 2025). This multimodal approach supports more informed and personalized decision-making in polytrauma care.

The image systems also have AI features that enhance communication between radiologists, surgeons and emergency doctors by creating organized reports and visual alerts. All these features simplify operations and deliver the most vital information to the decision-makers promptly. Altogether, AI is now an important supplement of trauma imaging, which helps increase the effectiveness of the diagnostic process and supports timely and data-driven clinical judgments in polytrauma.

9.7. AI in surgical decision-making and operative planning

One of the most complicated issues in the trauma care is surgical decision-making in polytrauma. The task of surgeons is to provide a balance between the immediate need to correct life-threatening injuries and consider the physiological reserves of the patient, a possible threat of complications and his or her overall prognosis. Conventional decision-making is based on clinical experience, intraoperative testing and physiological indicators, which differ among clinicians and intra-institutions. AI is currently offering an objective and specific aid to such decisions.

ML models are used to predict the survival, postoperative complications and the necessity to reoperate with patients who have polytrauma during surgery (Yang et al. 2020). These models are created by integrating such variables as pattern of injury, hemodynamic condition, laboratory results and imaging results, providing surgeons with a risk profile tailored to each patient to select the most appropriate operative approach. They particularly come in handy when determining the fitness of a patient to undergo early definitive surgery or require the use of damage-control surgery.

AI-based decision-support systems are also helpful in the process of operative planning by predicting the amount of blood loss to be expected, the length of the surgery and the requirements of resources such as transfusions and ICU beds (Yu et al. 2024). These forecasts enhance team preparedness and association between the surgeons, anesthesiologists and critical staff. In complicated cases where there are several injuries, AI systems can sort by the estimated physiological effects and survival value to select surgical procedures.

New reinforcement-learning strategies will improve the sequential decision-making in dynamic trauma situations of surgery. The systems with learning on past pairs of decisions and outcomes can propose adaptive strategies that change as the condition of the patient varies (Hasan et al. 2024). During surgery, AI-based monitoring is able to highlight possible instability at the early stages, enabling changes in approach or area to be made accordingly.

In sum, AI serves as an addition to the professional knowledge of surgeons to assist them during surgical decision-making in polytrauma by offering evidence-based, patient-specific information. The introduction of AI into the procedure of operative planning can make workflows less variable, safer and more productive in complicated trauma surgery.

9.8. AI in intensive care management of polytrauma

The polytrauma patient is a highly sensitive scenario in the ICU, and constant attention, immediate response and predictive decision-making are the key to avoiding the development of more complications and increasing survival.

Some of the common conditions that are experienced by the ICU patients are sepsis, acute respiratory distress syndrome, multi-organ failure and neurological deterioration. The onus of dealing with these changing situations imposes excessive cognitive load on clinicians. AI provides superior tools to aid ICU decision-making with the help of real-time analytics and predictive modeling.

The continuous physiological data necessary to analyze with AI-based monitoring devices are heart rate, blood pressure, oxygen saturation, intracranial pressure and ventilator settings. The field of DL (particularly RNNs) is especially good at identifying indications of deterioration early before the standard threshold alarms can be activated (Zace et al. 2025). Early warning systems based on AI allow early intervention, which lowers negative events.

Sepsis, ventilator-associated pneumonia and acute kidney injury are also complications that are predicted by ML (Danoe et al. 2024). Early identification of at-risk patients can enable selective monitoring, the initiation of the therapy and the effective distribution of resources, particularly in overcrowded ICUs that have limited personnel due to augmented decision support based on AI.

The AI systems assist in the decision on mechanical ventilation, fluid management and sedation, as they examine the patient-specific reactions to intervention. Adaptive algorithms prescribe the ventilator or fluid plan according to the evidence of anticipated results and help in personalized critical care (Peng et al. 2023). Data visualization aided by AI also helps to cut down on the workload of the clinicians because it displays complicated data in an intuitive way.

The involvement of AI in the management of ICUs leads to more situational awareness, uniformity and efficacy in the nursing care of critically ill polytrauma patients. AI contributes to safe and effective decision-making in the ICU by enhancing clinician judgment by providing continuous and data-driven insights.

9.9. Outcome prediction and prognostication using AI

There is a necessity to predict the results in cases of polytrauma. It will influence our decision-making, use of resources and the way we communicate to the families of the patients. The use of classic tools is beneficial, yet they rely on a limited number of variables and fixed snapshots and, therefore, might overlook the dynamic trajectory of the trauma physiology. The deep analysis of complex, multi-layered data enhances prognostication because AI generates personalized and constantly updated predictions.

ML models have become general place in predicting both short-term and long-term outcomes in polytrauma patients including death, hospital stay, ICU requirement and functional recovery (Alserhani 2025). They draw information on numerous sources, such as demographics, injury severity, vital, lab, imaging and treatments. The AI models are more accurate and flexible than the traditional ones.

DL techniques are effective for exploring nonlinear relations and time-dependent patterns. They can recalculate prognosis in real time by continually analyzing physiological time series to reflect changes in the state of a patient and his or her reaction to treatment (Lee et al. 2023). These dynamic updates will assist clinicians in making superior choices regarding whether to escalate or depress treatment.

Ethical and transparent decision-making using the AI-generated prediction is also encouraged through providing objective risk scores that can be discussed by the teams and families. These scores direct discussions on prognosis, care aspirations and rehabilitation plans, especially in case of severe brain damage issues or prolonged critical care (Choi et al. 2024).

Concisely, AI enhances predictive analytics in polytrauma by providing rapid, personal and evidence-based predictions. Such advantages enhance planning and optimization as well as support patient-centered decisions at every phase of trauma care. Table 9.1 contains AI applications categorized in the continuum of trauma care.

Stage of polytrauma care	AI techniques used	Key clinical decision-support functions	Primary clinical benefits
Prehospital Management	Machine learning, predictive analytics, wearable sensor analytics	Injury severity prediction, field triage optimization, transport destination selection	Reduced under-triage and over-triage, faster access to definitive trauma care
Emergency Department Triage	ML models, deep learning, NLP	Acuity prediction, early shock detection, prioritization of diagnostics	Improved triage accuracy, reduced time to intervention
Early Clinical Assessment	Time-series deep learning, NLP	Continuous risk reassessment, extraction of key clinical information	Reduced cognitive load, improved situational awareness
Imaging and Diagnostics	CNNs multimodal AI	Automated injury detection, severity quantification, report prioritization	Faster diagnosis, reduced inter-observer variability
Surgical Decision-Making	ML prediction models, reinforcement learning	Operative timing decisions, damage-control vs. definitive surgery selection	Optimized operative strategy, improved surgical outcomes
Operative Planning	Predictive analytics	Blood loss estimation, transfusion needs, ICU resource planning	Improved preparedness and resource utilization
Intensive Care Management	RNNs early warning systems	Deterioration detection, complication prediction (sepsis, AKI, ARDS)	Proactive intervention, reduced ICU morbidity
Outcome Prediction and Prognostication	ML and deep learning models	Mortality prediction, length of stay estimation, functional outcome forecasting	Improved clinical planning and family counseling
Ethical and Implementation Oversight	Explainable AI, federated learning	Bias mitigation, transparency, privacy preservation	Safer, fairer, and scalable AI deployment

Table 9.1. *Applications of AI across the continuum of polytrauma management*

9.10. Ethical, legal and implementation challenges of AI in polytrauma care

Although AI has tremendous potential in polytrauma decision-making, its application in clinics has ethical, legal and practical barriers. These challenges are critical to safe, just and effective use.

One of the ethical issues is algorithmic bias. The ML powering AI models is based on historical data, which can reproduce the disparity in the real world: age, sex, income or geography. Such biases may infiltrate and even intensify biased recommendations if they are not restrained, which is detrimental to fragile trauma patients (Moazemi et al. 2023). Between-subject training data is required.

Such issues as transparency and explainability are challenging. Most AI systems and particularly DL systems are black boxes, providing results without providing the steps taken to arrive at the result. Doctors in high-stakes polytrauma settings might be unwilling to put their faith in clouded advice. Explainable AI aims at fostering trust and accountability through increasing the clarity of outputs.

The question of legal and regulatory considerations is burdensome. It is not yet clear how there can be liability if an error in decision-making happens because of AI. The need to pin the blame on the doctors, hospitals and tech creators requires strong regulations on the issue and policies of governance. Privacy and security of data are also of high priority with delicate trauma information and increasing digital connectivity.

The application of AI into daily life is a difficult undertaking. To succeed, AI will have to be connected to the electronic health records (EHRs) without any hitches, integrate itself into the routine of clinicians and align with the current trauma regulations. Rollout can be slowed by resistance and lack of modern infrastructure and resources.

The comprehensive solution of such ethical, legal and practical issues is the key to realizing the full potential of AI in polytrauma care. The design must be created carefully, validated stringently and inter-disciplinary collaboration is necessary to ensure that AI will never harm patients and decision-making.

9.11. Future directions and emerging trends in AI-driven polytrauma decision-making

The future of AI in polytrauma lies in improved data fusion and the use of clear models and real-time implementation. AI will enhance the precision and speed of decisions, as well as personalization, since trauma care generates multifaceted, multimodal data.

One of these trends is the development of explainable AI systems providing transparent and understandable answers. The tools enhance trust, facilitate clinical validation and support shared decision-making because they demonstrate the main variables that lead to the results. Such clarity is particularly vital in high-risk trauma where the issue of accountability is crucial.

Another promising direction is federated learning. It enables model training across multiple locations without sharing raw patient data, addressing privacy concerns while developing more robust and generalizable models across diverse trauma populations. This approach can reduce institutional bias and improve the applicability of AI across different healthcare settings.

The use of AI in clinical support in real-time will increase. In the future, a combination of constant vital-sign tracking, screening of images and EHR will provide context-information-rich advice at the bedside.

Individual computing and wearables can also be used to allow AI to assist in making decisions in pre-hospital or low-resource environments.

Digital-twin models and reinforcement learning can also present simulation-based support, whereby the clinicians can experiment with treatment choices and preempt their consequences. These developments hold an improved approach to multifaceted and multiphase decisions in polytrauma management.

Further research, cross-disciplinary collaboration, and rigorous clinical validation are essential to translating emerging AI tools into safe, effective, and widely adopted decision support systems in polytrauma care.

9.12. Conclusion

Decision-making during polytrauma treatment is one of the most challenging tasks in modern healthcare. It requires rapid, accurate and synchronized operations in a state of unpredictability and strict schedules. Although traditional decision-making models are beneficial, they are frequently unable to deal with the influx of mixed data and are too slow to respond to the variations in patient conditions. This review demonstrates the way AI has become an influential support for clinicians, providing evidence-based assistance at every step of polytrauma treatment. AI enhances pre-hospital triage, ED evaluation, imaging tests, operation design, ICU care and patient results prediction. Through ML, DL and NLP, AI can identify complexities, predict degradation and recommend timely solutions in complex cases that would otherwise go unnoticed in an environment with high levels of stress. These strengths enhance accuracy, reduce variation in care and maximize use of important resources. Nevertheless, to enjoy the fruits of AI, we have to overcome ethical, legal and practical challenges. The issues of bias, transparency, data safety and the confidence of clinicians should be addressed by effective model design, testing and governance. Above all, AI should always be used as an addition to human judgment, as opposed to a substitution.

9.13. References

Adebayo, O., Bhuiyan, Z.A., Ahmed, Z. (2023). Exploring the effectiveness of artificial intelligence, machine learning and deep learning in trauma triage: A systematic review and meta-analysis. *Digital Health*, 9, 20552076231205736.

Alserhani, F. (2025). Intrusion detection and real-time adaptive security in medical IoT using a cyber-physical system design. *Sensors*, 25(15), 4720.

Baur, D., Gehlen, T., Scherer, J., Back, D.A., Tsitsilonis, S., Kabir, K., Osterhoff, G. (2022). Decision support by machine learning systems for acute management of severely injured patients: A systematic review. *Frontiers in Surgery*, 9, 924810.

Biswas, N., Ali, M.M., Rahaman, M.A., Islam, M., Mia, M.R., Azam, S., Ahmed, K., Bui, F.M., Al-Zahrani, F.A., Moni, M.A. (2023). Machine learning-based model to predict heart disease in early stage employing different feature selection techniques. *BioMed Research International*, 2023(1), 6864343.

Choi, A., Choi, S.Y., Chung, K., Chung, H.S., Song, T., Choi, B., Kim, J.H. (2023). Development of a machine learning-based clinical decision support system to predict clinical deterioration in patients visiting the emergency department. *Scientific Reports*, 13(1), 8561.

Choi, A., Lee, K., Hyun, H., Kim, K.J., Ahn, B., Lee, K.H., Hahn, S., Choi, S.Y., Kim, J.H. (2024). A novel deep learning algorithm for real-time prediction of clinical deterioration in the emergency department for a multimodal clinical decision support system. *Scientific Reports*, 14(1), 30116.

Danoe, G., Voss, A., Hamprecht, A., Berends, M.S. (2024). Artificial intelligence in infectious disease management: A scoping review of diagnostics, prognostics, modelling, surveillance, and forecasting. *SSRN Preprint*. doi: 10.2139/ssrn.5225402.

Hasan, R., Dattana, V., Mahmood, S., Hussain, S. (2024). Towards transparent diabetes prediction: Combining automl and explainable AI for improved clinical insights. *Information*, 16(1), 7.

Hunter, O.F., Perry, F., Salehi, M., Bandurski, H., Hubbard, A., Ball, C.G., Morad Hameed, S. (2023). Science fiction or clinical reality: A review of the applications of artificial intelligence along the continuum of trauma care. *World Journal of Emergency Surgery*, 18(1), 16.

Kang, W.S., Chung, H., Ko, H., Kim, N.Y., Kim, D.W., Cho, J., Shim, H., Kim, J.G., Jang, J.Y., Kim, K.W. et al. (2021). Artificial intelligence to predict in-hospital mortality using novel anatomical injury score. *Scientific Reports*, 11(1), 23534.

Lee, S., Kang, W.S., Seo, S., Kim, D.W., Ko, H., Kim, J., Lee, S., Lee, J. (2022). Model for predicting in-hospital mortality of physical trauma patients using artificial intelligence techniques: Nationwide population-based study in Korea. *Journal of Medical Internet Research*, 24(12), e43757.

Lee, S., Kang, W.S., Kim, D.W., Seo, S.H., Kim, J., Jeong, S.T., Yon, D.K., Lee, J. (2023). An artificial intelligence model for predicting trauma mortality among emergency department patients in South Korea: Retrospective cohort study. *Journal of Medical Internet Research*, 25, e49283.

Li, D., Xing, W., Zhao, J., Shi, C., Wang, F. (2025). Multimodal deep learning for predicting in-hospital mortality in heart failure patients using longitudinal chest X-rays and electronic health records. *The International Journal of Cardiovascular Imaging*, 41(3), 427–440.

Liu, Z., Huang, Y., Li, L., Xu, Y., Wu, P., Zhang, Z., Han, T., Zhang, L., Zhang, M. (2025). Development and clinical application of an automated machine learning-based delirium risk prediction model for emergency polytrauma patients. *Frontiers in Physiology*, 16, 1629329.

Mayerhoffer, H. and Ilić, B. (2025). Technological advancements in triage: How the development of artificial intelligence is changing medical practice – A literature review. *Croatian Nursing Journal*, 9(2), 279–302.

Moazemi, S., Vahdati, S., Li, J., Kalkhoff, S., Castano, L.J., Dewitz, B., Bibo, R., Sabouniaghdam, P., Tootooni, M.S., Bundschuh, R.A. et al. (2023). Artificial intelligence for clinical decision support for monitoring patients in cardiovascular ICUs: A systematic review. *Frontiers in Medicine*, 10, 1109411.

Peng, H.T., Siddiqui, M.M., Rhind, S.G., Zhang, J., da Luz, L.T., Beckett, A. (2023). Artificial intelligence and machine learning for hemorrhagic trauma care. *Military Medical Research*, 10(1), 6.

Rajaei, F., Cheng, S., Williamson, C.A., Wittrup, E., Najarian, K. (2023). AI-based decision support system for traumatic brain injury: A survey. *Diagnostics*, 13(9), 1640.

Swain, P. (2025). *The Artificial Intelligence and Machine Learning Blueprint: Foundations, Frameworks, and Real-World Applications*. Deep Science Publishing, Cambridge.

Toy, J., Warren, J., Wilhelm, K., Putnam, B., Whitfield, D., Gausche-Hill, M., Bosson, N., Donaldson, R., Schlesinger, S., Cheng, T. et al. (2024). Use of artificial intelligence to support prehospital traumatic injury care: A scoping review. *JACEP Open*, 5(5), e13251.

Ventura, C.A.I., Denton, E.E. and David, J.A. (2024). Artificial intelligence in emergency trauma care: A preliminary scoping review. *Medical Devices: Evidence and Research*, 17, 191–211. doi: 10.2147/MDER.S467146.

Xu, Y., Quan, R., Xu, W., Huang, Y., Chen, X., Liu, F. (2024). Advances in medical image segmentation: A comprehensive review of traditional, deep learning and hybrid approaches. *Bioengineering*, 11(10), 1034.

Yang, S., Yin, B., Cao, W., Feng, C., Fan, G., He, S. (2020). Diagnostic accuracy of deep learning in orthopaedic fractures: A systematic review and meta-analysis. *Clinical Radiology*, 75(9), 713-e17.

Yu, M., Wang, S., He, K., Teng, F., Deng, J., Guo, S., Yin, X., Lu, Q., Gu, W. (2024). Predicting the complexity and mortality of polytrauma patients with machine learning models. *Scientific Reports*, 14(1), 8302.

Zace, D., Semeraro, F., Schnaubelt, S., Montomoli, J., Ristagno, G., Fijačko, N., Gamberini, L., Bignami, E.G., Greif, R., Monsieurs, K.G., Scapigliati, A. (2025). Artificial intelligence in resuscitation: a scoping review. *Resuscitation Plus*, 24, 100973. doi: 10.1016/j.resplu.2025.100973.

Zhang, J., Contreras, M., Bandyopadhyay, S., Davidson, A., Sena, J., Ren, Y., Guan, Z., Ozrazgat-Baslanti, T., Loftus, T.J., Nerella, S. et al. (2024). MANGO: Multimodal Acuity Transformer for IntelliGent ICU Outcomes. *arXiv Preprint*, arXiv:2412.17832.

Zia, A., Fletcher, C., Bigwood, S., Ratnakanthan, P., Seah, J., Lee, R., Kavnoudias, H., Law, M. (2022). Retrospective analysis and prospective validation of an AI-based software for intracranial haemorrhage detection at a high-volume trauma centre. *Scientific Reports*, 12(1), 19885.

10

Outcome Prediction After Rotator Cuff Repair Using AI-Assisted Clinical Models

Rotator cuff repair is an orthopedic surgery that is widely used because it can stabilize the shoulder, recover its functionality and alleviate pain, but the postoperative outcomes of this procedure are not homogenous. Some of the variables that determine outcomes are the size of the tear, quality of the tissues, age, comorbid conditions, surgical method used and adherence rate of patients to the rehabilitation process. The conventional prediction tools (clinical scoring systems and regression models) are typically not accurate enough since they do not have the ability to capture the complex and nonlinear interactions between the multiple variables. Clinical models using artificial intelligence (AI) have been demonstrated to be promising in the past years to enhance outcome prediction following rotator cuff repair. These models incorporate infrequent, heterogeneous types of data, including clinical, imaging, surgical and rehab data, to predict tendon healing, risk of re-tear, pain intensity, functional recovery and suitability of revision surgery by using machine rather than deep-learning algorithms. They also have access to longitudinal data in terms of electronic health records and wearable sensors, thus enabling dynamic and personalized predictions. Irrespective of these benefits, data quality, model interpretability, external validation and ethical concerns remain a challenge that impedes clinical adoption. This chapter provides a critical review of existing AI-based prediction models used in rotator cuff repair, their techniques, advantages and drawbacks, and the possible clinical inference. In our synthesis, we will explain how AI applications can facilitate precision medicine, and enhance patient education and prevention in order to enhance and support postoperative care.

10.1. Introduction

Rotator cuff tears are a major cause of shoulder dysfunctions, pain and disability in most parts of the world, particularly in elderly people and individuals who are involved in monotonous overhead activities or

---

Chapter written by Vikas DESHMUKH and Prashant S. JADHAV.

occupations that involve repetitive and heavy physical jobs. Stabilization of the glenohumeral joint and achievement of smooth movement are the functions of the collaboration between the rotator cuff muscles supraspinatus, infraspinatus, subscapularis and teres minor, which depend on each other. Either degenerative or traumatic tendon injuries are capable of interfering with the mechanics of the shoulder, reducing its strength and making daily tasks (e.g. lifting, reaching, overhead motions) more difficult. Rotator cuff disease has a big socioeconomic impact in terms of financial expenditure on medical care, loss of work time and continued rehabilitation expenses, as well as productivity loss (Rodriguez et al. 2023; Routledge et al. 2023).

A rotator cuff tear is medically evaluated by surgery: it is a medical standard to use surgery as treatment of symptomatic rotator cuff tears that are unresponsive to conservative management, which includes physical therapy, activity change and medicine. Methods have changed to include open and mini-open procedures in modern arthroscopic repair, which are more preferable because of low invasiveness, less post-operative pain, faster recovery and higher cosmetic outcomes. In spite of such technical advances, recurring tear rates range between 10% and above 40%, and this depends on the size of tears, quality of tendons and chronicity, in addition to patient characteristics (Alaiti et al. 2023). Patients are not relieved of lingering pain, weakness or restricted mobility, even in cases where the repair has been structurally successful.

It is not easy to predict the results following rotator cuff repair due to the numerous factors that interrelate with the healing process and the process itself. Factors in patients such as age, sex and body mass index (BMI), and comorbidities such as diabetes, high cholesterol and smoking change the quality of tissue and blood supply, resulting in cellular repair issues (Routledge et al. 2023). Tear properties such as size, focalization, retraction, fatty infiltration and muscle shrinkage also interfere with structural and functional success. Chronic tears in particular pose a very big problem in that degenerative alterations lower the potential for healing and increase the possibility of failure (Alaiti et al. 2023). There is more variability in surgical variables, including repair technique, sutures, the number and location of anchors, tendon tension and the intra-operative quality of tissue. Finally, compliance with postoperation rehabilitation, including (controlled) mobilization, strengthening and functional exercises is also essential in ensuring good recovery.

Conventional methods for prediction, such as regression models and clinician judgments, find it hard to work with accuracy due to the inability to fully represent the nonlinear, multidimensional interactions between these variables. Linear and logistic regressions are based on a set of simple relationships; they are often based on the selection of features and do not consider the interactions among prognostic variables. Other problems that could affect the reliability and generalizability of any model include multicollinearity, unavailability of data and small samples of data (Niculescu 2020). Because of that, these traditional tools may not generate accurate and individualized predictions that can be used to inform clinical decision-making.

Artificial intelligence (AI) provides a disruptive solution in the medical field by learning the patterns based on received data to draw conclusions and assist with decision-making. Machine learning, an AI subset, enables algorithms to become better with the availability of more data without explicit programming. A further subsumption, known as deep learning, entails the use of multilayer neural networks, which automatically find complex components within unadjusted information such as imaging or time-series retail information (Niculescu 2020). These are the strengths of AI that make it particularly appropriate in outcome prediction during rotator cuff repair when multiple variables interacting with each other determine the postoperative trajectory.

Orthopedic studies have included machine-learning models (random forests, gradient-boosting machines, support vectors and k-nearest neighbors) to predict the surgical results, risk of complication and/or rehabilitation outcomes. Deep-learning algorithms and convolutional neural networks, in particular, have demonstrated a high level of accuracy in imaging (magnetic resonance imaging (MRI) and ultrasound) analysis, in terms of extracting quantitative features, such as tendon quality, fatty infiltration and muscle atrophy. The combination of several types of data allows AI-based models to make personalized predictions, which are more accurate than the traditional statistical models (Niculescu 2020).

The use of AI in rotator cuff repair is in accordance with the principles of precision-medicine, which provides the patient with personalized care according to their individual risk profile. The predictive models allow the stratification of patients based on re-tear risk, delayed functional recovery or persistent pain so that surgeons can modify methods, take into account biologic augmentation single-center or prescribe more serious rehab to high-risk patients. Minimal-risk patients can continue on through rehabilitation or can prematurely resume activity, which may lead to the reduction of healthcare costs and possibly shorten the recovery period. AI predictions empower shared decision-making as they also offer patients personalized prognostic data that can help them have realistic expectations and feel more satisfied.

Although AI has potential, a number of obstacles stem its extensive use. The interpretability of models is still a key issue that needs to be addressed. In order to use predictions effectively as part of the care, clinicians should be able to rely on explanations that are easy to understand. Most machine-learning and deep-learning algorithms are black boxes, which provide effective and correct predictions, but with no transparency. Other challenges to proposals are the quality of data, the lack of external validation and the penetration of the algorithms in clinical processes and ethics (patient privacy and algorithmic bias) that require consideration prior to regular use. To solve such issues, it is necessary to have strict methodology development, prospective multicenter research, explainable AI systems and intense cooperation between clinicians, data scientists and regulators (Kholinne et al. 2021).

10.2. Clinical outcomes after rotator cuff repair

Rotator cuff repair clinical outcomes are typically measured in three categories, such as structural, functional and patient-reported data. Structural data is based on the integrity of the tendon and its healing condition, which is examined by surgeons, using MRI or ultrasound, postoperatively. In its turn, good tendon healing implies stronger and more functional shoulders, whereas a failed tendon or a re-torn tendon is associated with poor outcomes (Kholinne et al. 2021). Nevertheless, a healthy tendon is not necessarily equal a contented and functional patient, as it has been demonstrated, which makes outcome assessment complex.

The objective measures of functional outcomes deal with shoulder range of motion, muscle strength and the performance of patients in their daily activities. Recovery is measured by common scoring systems, which include Constant Murley, American Shoulder and Elbow Surgeons, UCLA and the Simple Shoulder Test (Mosher et al. 2020). These tools can provide valuable information on functionality, but can easily be influenced by patient expectations and their subjective emotions.

Pain, perceived ability and general quality of life are needed since they are only assessed by the patient. The biggest element in patient satisfaction is often the relief of pain, even with minimal functional gains (Aagaard et al. 2023). Despite the numerous tools, postoperative outcomes cannot be predicted similarly. Such variation demonstrates that more effective prediction models (that are multicast integrals of clinical, imaging and patient individualized data) are required in decision-making and care delivery.

10.3. Limitations of conventional predictive models

The classical methods of health predicting the success of the procedure of rotator cuff repair involve simple statistical tools such as linear regression, logistic regression and survival analysis. They aid in the identification of the risk factors of poor healing or poor functioning, although their forecasts are not strong in daily practice. The fact that they assume a linear change in variables due to outcomes is one of the greatest shortcomings, as tendon biology and biomechanics do not change linearly with the results (Bartley 2021).

Other traditional models are also based on the pre-choice of features based on clinical know-how, which may overlook mere important interactions. The overlapping of variables such as age, tear size, muscle degeneration and such overlaps are termed as multicollinearity, and this makes builds tough and interpretations shaky. This makes the predictions inconsistent when using them on diversified groups of patients (Verma et al. 2021).

Another weakness is that most works rely on small and single-center datasets, which have limited power and generalizability. The analysis cannot address high-dimensional data such as imaging features or the finer metrics of rehab due to the limitation of analysis. Valuable information is thus wasted. It is against these issues that there has been interest in sophisticated ways to handle massive complex data and extrapolate nonlinear trends.

10.4. AI and ML in orthopedics

AI enables computer programs to carry out the functions that are traditionally performed by human intelligence, i.e. recognition of patterns, decisions and forecasting. Machine learning is a subdivision of AI that learns using data and gets better without any specific written instructions. A subset of machine learning is deep learning, which uses multi-layer neural networks to extract complex features of raw data automatically. These technologies have become popular in orthopedics due to the ability to handle large quantities of multi-dimensional data (Maffulli et al. 2020).

Algorithms such as support vector machines, random forests, gradient boosting machines and k-nearest neighbors have been used in orthopedic studies to predict outcomes, complications and readmissions. They are very good at nonlinearity between a large number of clinical variables (Feuerriegel et al. 2023). Convolutional neural networks and deep learning, in particular, have demonstrated great capability in imaging, being able to detect and classify tears of the rotator cuff from MRI and ultrasound images (Gillet et al. 2021).

Compared to traditional practices in orthopedic surgery, there are a number of advantages in using AI models. They are able to make more precise predictions, work with a larger amount of data, and combine multiple sources of data, including imaging, electronic health records and wearables. Accordingly, AI has been investigated in more and more cases to explain the post-rotator cuff repair outcome, which can be used to enhance counseling, surgical decisions or individualized rehabilitation studies.

10.5. Data sources for AI-assisted outcome prediction

Prediction models that are aided by AI are best applied to high-quality data, which is gathered by several sources. Most of the models have a clinical basis, and these include age, BMI, diabetes diagnosis, smoking habits, activity and shoulder baseline scores. These factors are predictable and affect the outcomes of post-operations, and are incorporated into most machine-learning algorithms (Rahmani et al. 2022).

Another important artwork is imaging. Pre-operational MRI gives meticulous causes and effects of tears, tendon retraction, muscle atrophy and fatty infiltration; all are good predictors of recovery and functionality. Deep learning is able to draw quantitative characteristics of images that a reader may not initially recognize (Kumar et al. 2025). The predictions can be fine-tuned with respect to the post-operative imaging to track tendon conditions.

The technique, type of fixation used, quantity of anchors and quality of tissue used can all provide prognostic information. Rehab data, including compliance with exercise plans and the progress of motion, are now measured through digital devices and wearables. Connecting electronic health records enables constant monitoring of results and complications, which enables AI to make predictions that may be changed and tailored to patients and their recovery (Shinohara et al. 2024).

10.6. AI models for predicting tendon healing and re-tear risk

It is essential to determine the healing of tendons and their vulnerable state in terms of re-tear. The causes of structural failure can also lead to persistent pain, bad shoulders and lack of functionality.

Based on its prediction of these outcomes, AI models demonstrate the potent approach to integrating pre-operative clinical data, imaging and surgical factors. Random forests, support vector machines and boosting models also perform better than the old-fashioned regression in identifying patients with a high risk of re-tear (Kang et al. 2021).

Convolutional neural networks and, more broadly, the field of deep learning are becoming important to preoperative MRI analysis. Such models automatically identify features that are associated with tendon quality, muscle loss and fatty infiltration, which are difficult to measure. It has been demonstrated that deep-learning imaging analysis is highly sensitive and specific in forecasting healing compared to the traditional radiology presentation (Campagnini et al. 2022).

AI models can also assist clinicians in categorizing risk as low, medium and high in the case of structural failure. The latter informs pre-operative choices based on the type of surgery, bio-augmentation or changes to rehab regimens. Results are promising, but there are numerous works that are retrospective and not externalized. These models require continuous development and validation in diverse patients before they can be considered a useful tool in routine practice.

10.7. Prediction of functional recovery and pain outcomes

Although structural integrity is a worthy predictor of success post-rotator cuff repair, patients tend to be more interested in functional recovery and pain relief. The clinical models on AI-assisted prediction of the functioning and pain trend post-surgery are actively used to predict the functionality and pain of patients successfully in the future. These models take into consideration a great number of patient-specific variables. The performance of machine-learning algorithms using baseline functional scores, psychosocial factors and rehabilitation adherence, combined with tear characteristics, is higher than that of the baseline statistical approach (Sharma et al. 2024).

Rotator cuff repair requires both biological recovery and neuromuscular adaptation in order to achieve functional recovery. AI models are able to capture multifaceted relationships among pre-operative levels of shoulder functionality, muscle strength, range of movement and motivations of the patients. This will enable them to make better predictions of post-operative performance. The predictive models approximate post-operative scores on popular outcome scales, which include the American Shoulder and Elbow Surgeons score and the Constant Murley Score, helping the clinicians to establish achievable recovery outcomes (Chen et al. 2020).

The effect of post-operative pain is multifaceted. It depends on the factors in surgical procedures, inflammation, psychology and rehabilitation. AI methods are capable of forecasting protracted pain or delayed pain solutions. The satisfaction and quality of care received at the end of rotator cuff repair are better with early detection of patients who may require further and more effective pain management.

10.8. Integration of wearable and rehabilitation data

New methods of improving the predictability of outcomes of rotator cuff repair include the development of wearable technologies and digital rehabilitation systems. Wearable sensors that could continuously monitor shoulder movement, range of motion, activity of the shoulder or compliance with a given exercise, such as inertial measurement unit sensors and activity monitors can help monitor this. This data gives objective and high-resolution information on recovery that cannot be obtained by regular visits to the clinic (Papadopoulos et al. 2024).

AI models are fast at analyzing wearable data comprising large amounts of time-series data volumes. Machine-learning programs find functional patterns of recovery, anomalies in predicted patterns and prognosticate future long-term functional dynamics using initial post-surgical performance. With wearable metrics combined with clinical and imaging data, AI models lead to dynamic prediction that changes during rehabilitation (Lam et al. 2022).

Integrating rehabilitation data in use by AI adds to predictions and assists in customized and dynamic plans. Slow-progressing patients are likely to respond to modified exercise programs, extra physiotherapy or closer clinical supervision. On the contrary, faster-healing patients can safely proceed to exercises of higher stages sooner. Nonetheless, they still have a problem related to standardizing data, patient behavior and incorporating it into current processes. The need to handle those issues is how the clinical utility of wearable-informed prediction systems can be maximized.

10.9. Model performance and validation

The models that are supported by AI tend to perform better than the traditional statistical ones to predict outcomes following a rotator cuff repair. Numerous studies complain about increased accuracy, sensitivity, specificity and area under the receiver operating characteristic (ROC) curve using machine-learning and deep-learning models on more complicated clinical data (Wand et al. 2021). These benefits are due to the capability of AI algorithms to simulate nonlinear relationships and interactions of various predictors such as imaging features and longitudinal rehabilitation information.

Although the metrics used are promising, the question of validation is very important. Countless research is based on retrospective datasets in individual institutions, and this exposes them to overfitting as well as decreasing generally representative efficacy. Internal validation methods such as the use of cross-validation are frequently used, whereas external validation using independent multi-centric data are very few (Saraswat et al. 2022). The external validation of AI-assisted models is weak, and it is not clear how reliable the models will be in clinical settings.

A second limitation is the inability to have standardized outcome definitions and performance measures in the literature. These differences in outcome measures, duration of follow-up and standards of evaluation make it difficult to compare models and synthesize evidence. The applicability of the clinical transfer and standardization of reporting guidelines and transparent development practices are also likely to enhance reproducibility and enable clinical translation. Prospective validation and real-world testing should be a priority in future research so as to determine the effectiveness and safety in a normal orthopedic practice. The AI-assisted models of outcome prediction after rotator cuff repair can be found in Table 10.1.

Outcome domain	**Input data sources**	**AI/ML techniques used**	**Predicted clinical outcomes**	**Clinical utility**
Tendon Healing and Re-tear Risk	Clinical variables, MRI features (tear size, fatty infiltration), surgical parameters	Random forests, SVM, gradient boosting, CNNs	Tendon integrity, probability of re-tear	Risk stratification, surgical planning, biological augmentation decisions
Functional Recovery	Baseline functional scores, demographics, tear characteristics, rehab data	Machine learning regression models, ensemble learning	ASES score, Constant–Murley score, ROM recovery	Expectation setting, tailored rehabilitation intensity
Postoperative Pain Outcomes	Clinical data, psychosocial factors, rehabilitation adherence	ML classifiers, predictive analytics	Persistent pain, delayed pain resolution	Early pain-management intervention
Rehabilitation Progress	Wearable sensor data, activity tracking, time-series rehab metrics	Time-series ML, deep learning models	Recovery trajectory, deviation from expected progress	Adaptive and personalized rehabilitation protocols
Revision Surgery Risk	Combined clinical, imaging and outcome data	ML risk prediction models	Likelihood of revision surgery	Long-term follow-up planning and counseling
Longitudinal Outcome Forecasting	EHR data, imaging, wearable data	Multimodal AI, dynamic prediction models	Personalized, evolving outcome predictions	Precision medicine–driven postoperative management

Table 10.1. *AI-assisted models for outcome prediction after rotator cuff repair*

10.10. Interpretability and clinical acceptance

Although AI-assisted models have predictive advantages, their applicability is limited by low interpretability, which prevents common orthopedic usage. Neural networks are considered complex, and they work as black boxes, which do not explain explicitly what kinds of inputs affect the output. This non-transparency may negatively impact clinician trust and adoption, particularly in surgical choices that have high stakes (Molnar 2020).

The interpretation needs to be accepted by clinics. Surgeons must have clear reasons about why pre-surgical counseling and joint decision-making are necessary. The newest trends in explainable AI overcome this issue by emphasizing the value of individual predictors or visualizing the ways to input influence predictions. Methods such as feature importance ranking, saliency maps and local explanation methods have enhanced interpretability in orthopedic studies (Boudi et al. 2024).

Between interpretability and practical considerations, there are issues of acceptability. The convenience of fitting into existing workflows, efficiency and ability to integrate with electronic health records are important. AI tools that are easily integrated into daily care and offer implementable knowledge are more accepted. AI concepts, education and training instill more confidence in the proper use of predictive models. To achieve successful outcome prediction with the help of AI in rotator cuff repair, it is necessary to address the challenges of interpretability and usability.

10.11. Ethical, legal and practical considerations

The use of AI-aided prediction systems in rotator cuff repair creates various ethical, legal and practical concerns that need to be resolved prior to the implementation of the system. The privacy and security of data are significant issues since AI models are dependent on massive amounts of patient information in electronic health records, imaging databases and wearables. In order to foster trust, regulations concerning the protection of data and patient confidentiality are needed (Meszaros et al. 2022).

The other notable challenge is algorithmic bias. Unless the training data are reflective of different populations, the AI models can result in varying predictions that are harmful to some population groups. This kind of bias may exacerbate the situation of inequality and compromise equitable care. These risks require rigorous curation of datasets, bias auditing and constant monitoring of models to reduce such risks and have a fair performance across populations (Sisodiya 2021).

Law-wise, accountability and liability get cumbersome in cases where AI-assisted models affect clinical decisions. It is difficult to say who is responsible when wrong predictions or other bad results are made, and AI suggestions are processed in surgical planning or rehabilitation. Some of the practical issues include the costs of implementing it, the infrastructure requirements and the training necessary for the clinicians. The ethical, legal and operational concerns mentioned in this chapter are important in order to implement AI-assisted outcome prediction models into orthopedic practice in a responsible and sustainable way.

10.12. Future directions

The next generation of AI-based outcome prediction following rotator cuff repair should improve the robustness, generalizability and clinical utility of the model. Creating massive, multi-center and prospective data with varying patient groups and in different surgery and rehabilitation programs is among the top priorities. These statistics will reduce bias, enhance external validity and aid in the creation of more dependable predictive models (Ramgopal et al. 2023).

Another major avenue is that of data integration. The incorporation of new sources such as genomic data, biochemical measures of tendon healing and patient-reported experience measures would increase predictive accuracy. Multimodal AI models can be used to integrate clinical, imaging, biological and behavioral data, and offer holistic outcome prognosis. Furthermore, real-time adaptive postoperative control may be possible on the basis of continuous learning systems that update the predictions with new information.

To achieve clinical adoption, it is necessary to make models understandable and easy to use. The next-generation AI tools must provide understandable and practical information rather than isolated risk scores so that clinicians can modify the surgery and rehabilitation regimen. The intellectualized electronic health records may be packaged by embedding an intelligent prediction algorithm into the clinical decision-support systems, rendering them a normal procedure. It is important to continue working on this collaboration between clinicians, data scientists and regulators to ensure that AI developments would remain consistent with clinical requirements and ethical standards.

10.13. Implications for precision medicine

Outcome prediction using AI post-rotator cuff repair is well aligned with precision medicine, which deals with individually directed treatment. With a combination of clinical data, image characteristics, rehabilitation measurements and behavioral issues, AI models will be able to better sort patients by the likelihood of risk and rehabilitation pattern (Yogeshappa 2024).

Accurate prediction of results enables clinicians to provide personalized care to patients. High-risk patients with a risk of re-tear or slower recovery can get changed surgery, biological augmentation or more rigorous and highly monitored rehabilitation. Accelerated rehab protocols may reduce costs and time without negatively impacting outcomes by use in low-risk patients.

Shared decision-making is also reinforced in AI-assisted precision medicine since patients will receive personalized prognosis. Individual risk and anticipated results would be effectively communicated with the enhancement of understanding, setting reasonable expectations and increasing patient satisfaction. With the further development of AI, its implementation in the field of precision medicine would redefine the nature of post-operative support labor related to rotator cuff repair, as the use of a one-size-fits-all method is phased out and replaced by more patient-centered and data-driven solutions.

10.14. Conclusion

The use of AI-driven clinical models is one of the significant steps in outcome prediction following rotator cuff repair. AI is able to combine clinical data with imaging data, and surgical data with rehab data to achieve complex interactions that are impervious to traditional statistics. Such models are more accurate in forecasting tendon healing, risk of re-tear, functional recovery and pain, which justify individualization of risk stratification and specific post-operative care. The implementation of AI would improve precision medicine, shared decision-making and rehab planning, which will eventually improve the outcomes. However, there are still difficulties, which include interpretability, external validation, ethics and workflow integration. The identified issues require addressing future, multicentric research, standard reporting and explainable AI to mitigate the risk and adopt it safely and effectively.

10.15. References

Aagaard, K.E., Lunsjö, K., Adolfsson, L., Frobell, R., Hallgren, H.B. (2023). Factors associated with healing failure after early repair of acute, trauma-related rotator cuff tears. *Journal of Shoulder and Elbow Surgery*, 32(10), 2074–2081.

Alaiti, R.K., Vallio, C.S., Assunção, J.H., Andrade e Silva, F.B., Gracitelli, M.E., Neto, A.A., Malavolta, E.A. (2023). Using machine learning to predict nonachievement of clinically significant outcomes after rotator cuff repair. *Orthopaedic Journal of Sports Medicine*, 11(10), 23259671231206180.

Alanazi, A. (2022). Using machine learning for healthcare challenges and opportunities. *Informatics in Medicine Unlocked*, 30, 100924.

Bartley, A. (2021). Predictive analytics in healthcare. White Paper on Healthcare Predictive Analytics, Intel Corporation.

Boudi, A.L., Boudi, M., Chan, C., Boudi, F.B., Boudi, A. (2024). Ethical challenges of artificial intelligence in medicine. *Cureus*, 16(11).

Campagnini, S., Arienti, C., Patrini, M., Liuzzi, P., Mannini, A., Carrozza, M.C. (2022). Machine learning methods for functional recovery prediction and prognosis in post-stroke rehabilitation: A systematic review. *Journal of NeuroEngineering and Rehabilitation*, 19(1), 54.

Chen, Y.P., Lin, C.Y., Tsai, M.J., Chuang, T.Y., Lee, O.K. (2020). Wearable motion sensor device to facilitate rehabilitation in patients with shoulder adhesive capsulitis: Pilot study to assess feasibility. *Journal of Medical Internet Research*, 22(7), e17032.

Feuerriegel, G.C., Weiss, K., Kronthaler, S., Leonhardt, Y., Neumann, J., Wurm, M., Lenhart, N.S., Makowski, M.R., Schwaiger, B.J., Woertler, K. et al. (2023). Evaluation of a deep learning-based reconstruction method for denoising and image enhancement of shoulder MRI in patients with shoulder pain. *European Radiology*, 33(7), 4875–4884.

Gillet, R., Zhu, F., Padoin, P., Rauch, A., Hossu, G., Teixeira, P.A., Blum, A. (2021). MR imaging biomarkers for clinical impairment and disease progression in patients with shoulder adhesive capsulitis: A prospective study. *Journal of Clinical Medicine*, 10(17), 3882.

Kang, Y., Choi, D., Lee, K.J., Oh, J.H., Kim, B.R., Ahn, J.M. (2021). Evaluating subscapularis tendon tears on axillary lateral radiographs using deep learning. *European Radiology*, 31(12), 9408–9417.

Kholinne, E., Kwak, J.M., Cho, C.H., AlSomali, K., Van Nguyen, T., Kim, H., Koh, K.H., Jeon, I.H. (2021). Arthroscopic superior capsular reconstruction for older patients with irreparable rotator cuff tears: A comparative study with younger patients. *The American Journal of Sports Medicine*, 49(10), 2751–2759.

Kumar, A., Batta, P., Rathore, P.S., Ahuja, S. (2025). Secure healthcare data sharing and attack detection framework using radial basis neural network. *Scientific Reports*, 15(1), 15432.

Lam, K., Chen, J., Wang, Z., Iqbal, F.M., Darzi, A., Lo, B., Purkayastha, S., Kinross, J.M. (2022). Machine learning for technical skill assessment in surgery: A systematic review. *NPJ Digital Medicine*, 5(1), 24.

Maffulli, N., Rodriguez, H.C., Stone, I.W., Nam, A., Song, A., Gupta, M., Alvarado, R., Ramon, D., Gupta, A. (2020). Artificial intelligence and machine learning in orthopedic surgery: A systematic review protocol. *Journal of Orthopaedic Surgery and Research*, 15(1), 478.

Meszaros, J., Minari, J., Huys, I. (2022). The future regulation of artificial intelligence systems in healthcare services and medical research in the European Union. *Frontiers in Genetics*, 13, 927721.

Molnar, C. (2020). *Interpretable Machine Learning*. Lulu, Morisville, NC.

Mosher, Z.A., Ewing, M.A., Collins, C.S., Young, P.G., Brabston, E.W., Momaya, A.M., Tashjian, R.Z., Ponce, B.A. (2020). Usage trends of patient-reported outcome measures in shoulder literature. *JAAOS – Journal of the American Academy of Orthopaedic Surgeons*, 28(17), e774–e781.

Niculescu, V. (2020). On the impact of high performance computing in big data analytics for medicine. *Applied Medical Informatics*, 42(1), 9–18.

Papadopoulos, P., Soflano, M., Connolly, T. (2024). A digital health intervention platform (active and independent management system) to enhance the rehabilitation experience for orthopedic joint replacement patients: Usability evaluation study. *JMIR Human Factors*, 11, e50430.

Rahmani, A.M., Szu-Han, W., Yu-Hsuan, K., Haghparast, M. (2022). The internet of things for applications in wearable technology. *IEEE Access*, 10, 123579–123594.

Ramgopal, S., Sanchez-Pinto, L.N., Horvat, C.M., Carroll, M.S., Luo, Y., Florin, T.A. (2023). Artificial intelligence-based clinical decision support in pediatrics. *Pediatric Research*, 93(2), 334–341.

Rodriguez, H.C., Rust, B., Hansen, P.Y., Maffulli, N., Gupta, M., Potty, A.G., Gupta, A. (2023). Artificial intelligence and machine learning in rotator cuff tears. *Sports Medicine and Arthroscopy Review*, 31(3), 67–72.

Routledge, J.C., Saber, A.Y., Pennington, N., Gupta, N. (2023). Re-tear rates following rotator cuff repair surgery. *Cureus*, 15(1), e34426.

Saraswat, D., Bhattacharya, P., Verma, A., Prasad, V.K., Tanwar, S., Sharma, G., Bokoro, P.N., Sharma, R. (2022). Explainable AI for healthcare 5.0: Opportunities and challenges. *IEEE Access*, 10, 84486–84517.

Sharma, V., Mahajan, S., Zaki, M.H., Guria, S.N., Swathy, K., Sharma, M. (2024). AI-guided rehabilitation for stroke patients. In *4th International Conference on Advancement in Electronics & Communication Engineering (AECE)*, 22 November, 225–230. IEEE.

Shinohara, I., Mifune, Y., Inui, A., Nishimoto, H., Yoshikawa, T., Kato, T., Furukawa, T., Tanaka, S., Kusunose, M., Hoshino, Y. et al. (2024). Re-tear after arthroscopic rotator cuff tear surgery: Risk analysis using machine learning. *Journal of Shoulder and Elbow Surgery*, 33(4), 815–822.

Sisodiya, S.M. (2021). Precision medicine and therapies of the future. *Epilepsia*, 62, S90–S105.

Verma, A.A., Murray, J., Greiner, R., Cohen, J.P., Shojania, K.G., Ghassemi, M., Straus, S.E., Pou-Prom, C., Mamdani, M. (2021). Implementing machine learning in medicine. *CMAJ*, 193(34), E1351–E1357.

Wand, H., Lambert, S.A., Tamburro, C., Iacocca, M.A., O'Sullivan, J.W., Sillari, C., Kullo, I.J., Rowley, R., Dron, J.S., Brockman, D. et al. (2021). Improving reporting standards for polygenic scores in risk prediction studies. *Nature*, 591(7849), 211–219.

Yogeshappa, V.G. (2024). AI-driven precision medicine: Revolutionizing personalized treatment plans. *International Journal of Computer Engineering and Technology (IJCET)*, 15(5), 455–474.

List of Authors

Pisal Rutuja A.
Department of Mechanical Engineering
Jaywant College of Engineering and Polytechnic
Killemachindragadh
India

Priya BATTA
Amity School of Engineering and Technology
Amity University Punjab
Mohali
India

Piyush Ashokrao DALKE
Department of Mechanical Engineering
Shri Sant Gajanan Maharaj College of Engineering
Shegaon
India

Vikas DESHMUKH
Department of Orthopedics
Krishna Institute of Medical Sciences
Krishna Vishwa Vidyapeeth
"Deemed to be University"
Taluka-Karad
India

Amol S. DHAWALE
Department of Orthopedics
Krishna Institute of Medical Sciences
Krishna Vishwa Vidyapeeth
"Deemed to be University"
Taluka-Karad
India

Dalavi Surekha GORAKH
Department of Mechanical Engineering
Jaywant College of Engineering and Polytechnic
Killemachindragadh
India

Prashant S. JADHAV
Rajarambapu Institute of Technology
Shivaji University
Kolhapur
India

Jineshwar KAPALE
Department of Orthopedics
Krishna Institute of Medical Sciences
Krishna Vishwa Vidyapeeth
"Deemed to be University"
Taluka-Karad
India

Anupam S. KOLEKAR
Department of Orthopedics
Krishna Institute of Medical Sciences
Krishna Vishwa Vidyapeeth
"Deemed to be University"
Taluka-Karad
India

P.N. KULKARNI
Department of Orthopedics
Krishna Institute of Medical Sciences
Krishna Vishwa Vidyapeeth
"Deemed to be University"
Taluka-Karad
India

Abhishek KUMAR
Department of Computer Science and Engineering
Chandigarh University
Mohali
India

Attar Tabassum M.
Department of Mechanical Engineering
Jaywant College of Engineering and Polytechnic
Killemachindragadh
India

Channapa MAHAJAN
Department of Orthopedics
Krishna Institute of Medical Sciences
Krishna Vishwa Vidyapeeth
"Deemed to be University"
Taluka-Karad
India

More Seema NITIN
Department of Mechanical Engineering
Jaywant College of Engineering and Polytechnic
Killemachindragadh
India

Paresh PATIL
Department of Orthopedics
Krishna Institute of Medical Sciences
Krishna Vishwa Vidyapeeth
"Deemed to be University"
Taluka-Karad
India

Sandip R. PATIL
Department of Orthopedics
Krishna Institute of Medical Sciences
Krishna Vishwa Vidyapeeth
"Deemed to be University"
Taluka-Karad
India

Santosh TAKALE
Department of Orthopedics
Krishna Institute of Medical Sciences
Krishna Vishwa Vidyapeeth
"Deemed to be University"
Taluka-Karad
India

Chavan Vikrant U.
Department of Mechanical Engineering
Jaywant College of Engineering and Polytechnic
Killemachindragadh
India

Index

M, N

P

R, S

T, U, W

Other titles from

iSTE

in

Computer Engineering

2026

BHAMBRI Pankaj, DUTTA Pushan Kumar, KHAN Mudassir, STAROSTKA-PATYK Marta
Next-Gen Supply Chains: AI, Automation, and Sustainability in a Disrupted World

DARCHE Philippe
Computer Memories 1: Core Concepts
Computer Memories 2: Static Random-Access Memory

KUMAR Abhishek, BATTA Priya, AHUJA Sachin, RATHORE Pramod Singh
AI-driven Innovations in Physiotherapy and Oncology 3

KUMAR Abhishek, BATTA Priya, ANANTH J.P.
AI-driven Healthcare Innovations: Applications in Neurology and Medicine

MACHADO Carolina, DAVIM J. Paulo
Artificial Intelligence Technologies in Management and Engineering

MAHOUT Vincent, ROCACHER Thierry, AURIOL Guillaume
Programming of Embedded Systems: Applications to SM32F10x μControllers

2025

CHIKH Azeddine
Systemic Approach to Categorizing and Modeling Requirements

KUMAR Abhishek, BATTA Priya, AHUJA Sachin,
RATHORE Pramod Singh
AI-driven Innovations in Physiotherapy and Oncology 1
AI-driven Innovations in Physiotherapy and Oncology 2

TANEJA Ashu, KUMAR Abhishek, LIMKAR Suresh Vishnudas,
OUAISSA Mariya, OUAISSA Mariyam
Driving Innovation through AI and Digital Twin for 6G Powered Sustainable Ultra Smart Cities

TANEJA Ashu, KUMAR Abhishek, LIMKAR Suresh Vishnudas,
OUAISSA Mariya, OUAISSA Mariyam
6G Urban Innovation: AI and Digital Twin for Next-Gen Sustainable Cities

2024

CHAKRABORTY Rajdeep, GHOSH Anupam, KUMAR MANDAL Jyotsna,
CHOUDHURY Tanupriya, CHATTERJEE Prasenjit
Smart Edge Computing: An Operation Research Perspective
(International Perspectives in Decision Analytics and Operations Research Set – Volume 2)

HOMÈS Bernard
Fundamentals of Software Testing (2nd edition, revised and updated)

JERBI Abdessalem
Discrete-Event Simulation: Concepts and Production in Arena

PRADHAN Devasis, KUMAR SAHU Prasanna, MYO TUN Hla,
CHATTERJEE Prasenjit
Artificial and Cognitive Computing for Sustainable Healthcare Systems in Smart Cities
(International Perspectives in Decision Analytics and Operations Research Set – Volume 3)

2023

CHOUDHURY Tanupriya, KHANNA Abhirup, CHATTERJEE Prasenjit, UM Jung-Sup, BHATTACHARYA Abhishek
Blockchain Applications in Healthcare: Innovations and Practices (International Perspectives in Decision Analytics and Operations Research Set – Volume 1)

PAI G A Vijayalakshmi
A Textbook of Data Structures and Algorithms 1: Mastering Linear Data Structures
A Textbook of Data Structures and Algorithms 2: Mastering Nonlinear Data Structures
A Textbook of Data Structures and Algorithms 3: Mastering Advanced Data Structures and Algorithm Design Strategies

2022

HOMÈS Bernard
Advanced Testing of Systems-of-Systems 1: Theoretical Aspects
Advanced Testing of Systems-of-Systems 2: Practical Aspects

MEHTA Shikha, TIWARI Sanju, SIARRY Patrick, JABBAR M.A.
Tools, Languages, Methodologies for Representing Semantics on the Web of Things

SIDHOM Sahbi, KADDOUR Amira
Systems and Uses of Digital Sciences for Knowledge Organization (Digital Tools and Uses Set – Volume 9)

ZAIDOUN Ameur Salem
Computer Science Security: Concepts and Tools

2021

DARCHE Philippe
Microprocessor 4: Core Concepts – Software Aspects
Microprocessor 5: Software and Hardware Aspects of Development, Debugging and Testing – The Microcomputer

DELHAYE Jean-Loïc
Inside the World of Computing: Technologies, Uses, Challenges

HARDIN Thérèse, JAUME Mathieu, PESSAUX François,
VIGUIÉ DONZEAU-GOUGE Véronique
Concepts and Semantics of Programming Languages 1: A Semantical Approach with OCaml and Python
Concepts and Semantics of Programming Languages 2: Modular and Object-oriented Constructs with OCaml, Python, C++, Ada and Java

MKADMI Abderrazak
Archives in The Digital Age: Preservation and the Right to be Forgotten (Digital Tools and Uses Set – Volume 8)

TOKLU Yusuf Cengiz, BEKDAŞ Gebrail, NIGDELI Sinan Melih
Metaheuristics for Structural Design and Analysis (Optimization Heuristics Set – Volume 3)

2020

DARCHE Philippe
Microprocessor 1: Prolegomenes – Calculation and Storage Functions – Models of Computation and Computer Architecture
Microprocessor 2: Core Concepts – Communication in a Digital System
Microprocessor 3: Core Concepts – Hardware Aspects

DUVAUT Patrick, DALLOZ Xavier, MENGA David, KOEHL François,
CHRIQUI Vidal, BRILL Joerg
Internet of Augmented Me, I.AM: Empowering Innovation for a New Sustainable Future

LAFFLY Dominique
TORUS 1 – Toward an Open Resource Using Services: Cloud Computing for Environmental Data
TORUS 2 – Toward an Open Resource Using Services: Cloud Computing for Environmental Data
TORUS 3 – Toward an Open Resource Using Services: Cloud Computing for Environmental Data

LAURENT Anne, LAURENT Dominique, MADERA Cédrine
Data Lakes
(Databases and Big Data Set – Volume 2)

OULHADJ Hamouche, DAACHI Boubaker, MENASRI Riad
Metaheuristics for Robotics
(Optimization Heuristics Set – Volume 2)

SADIQUI Ali
Computer Network Security

VENTRE Daniel
Artificial Intelligence, Cybersecurity and Cyber Defense

2019

BESBES Walid, DHOUIB Diala, WASSAN Niaz, MARREKCHI Emna
Solving Transport Problems: Towards Green Logistics

CLERC Maurice
Iterative Optimizers: Difficulty Measures and Benchmarks

GHLALA Riadh
Analytic SQL in SQL Server 2014/2016

TOUNSI Wiem
Cyber-Vigilance and Digital Trust: Cyber Security in the Era of Cloud Computing and IoT

2018

ANDRO Mathieu
Digital Libraries and Crowdsourcing
(Digital Tools and Uses Set – Volume 5)

ARNALDI Bruno, GUITTON Pascal, MOREAU Guillaume
Virtual Reality and Augmented Reality: Myths and Realities

CARDON Alain
Beyond Artificial Intelligence: From Human Consciousness to Artificial Consciousness

HOMAYOUNI S. Mahdi, FONTES Dalila B.M.M.
Metaheuristics for Maritime Operations
(Optimization Heuristics Set – Volume 1)

JEANSOULIN Robert
JavaScript and Open Data

PIVERT Olivier
NoSQL Data Models: Trends and Challenges
(Databases and Big Data Set – Volume 1)

SEDKAOUI Soraya
Data Analytics and Big Data

SALEH Imad, AMMI Mehdi, SZONIECKY Samuel
Challenges of the Internet of Things: Technology, Use, Ethics
(Digital Tools and Uses Set – Volume 7)

SZONIECKY Samuel
Ecosystems Knowledge: Modeling and Analysis Method for Information and Communication
(Digital Tools and Uses Set – Volume 6)

2017

BENMAMMAR Badr
Concurrent, Real-Time and Distributed Programming in Java: Threads, RTSJ and RMI

BOUHAÏ Nasreddine, SALEH Imad
Internet of Things: Evolutions and Innovations
(Digital Tools and Uses Set – Volume 4)

HÉLIODORE Frédéric, NAKIB Amir, ISMAIL Boussaad, OUCHRAA Salma, SCHMITT Laurent
Metaheuristics for Intelligent Electrical Networks
(Metaheuristics Set – Volume 10)

MA Haiping, SIMON Dan
Evolutionary Computation with Biogeography-based Optimization
(Metaheuristics Set – Volume 8)

PÉTROWSKI Alain, BEN-HAMIDA Sana
Evolutionary Algorithms
(Metaheuristics Set – Volume 9)

PAI G A Vijayalakshmi
Metaheuristics for Portfolio Optimization: An Introduction using MATLAB®
(Metaheuristics Set – Volume 11)

REYES-GARCIA Everardo
The Image-Interface: Graphical Supports for Visual Information
(Digital Tools and Uses Set – Volume 3)

REYES-GARCIA Everardo, BOUHAÏ Nasreddine
Designing Interactive Hypermedia Systems
(Digital Tools and Uses Set – Volume 2)

SZONIECKY Samuel, BOUHAÏ Nasreddine
Collective Intelligence and Digital Archives: Towards Knowledge Ecosystems
(Digital Tools and Uses Set – Volume 1)

2016

BLUM Christian, FESTA Paola
Metaheuristics for String Problems in Bio-informatics
(Metaheuristics Set – Volume 6)

DEROUSSI Laurent
Metaheuristics for Logistics
(Metaheuristics Set – Volume 4)

DHAENENS Clarisse, JOURDAN Laetitia
Metaheuristics for Big Data
(Metaheuristics Set – Volume 5)

LABADIE Nacima, PRINS Christian, PRODHON Caroline
Metaheuristics for Vehicle Routing Problems
(Metaheuristics Set – Volume 3)

LEROY Laure
Eyestrain Reduction in Stereoscopy

LUTTON Evelyne, PERROT Nathalie, TONDA Alberto
Evolutionary Algorithms for Food Science and Technology
(Metaheuristics Set – Volume 7)

MAGOULÈS Frédéric, ZHAO Hai-Xiang
Data Mining and Machine Learning in Building Energy Analysis

RIGO Michel
Advanced Graph Theory and Combinatorics

ZELM Martin, DOUMEINGTS Guy, MENDONÇA Joao Pedro
Enterprise Interoperability: in the Digitized and Networked Factory of the Future

2015

BARBIER Franck, RECOUSSINE Jean-Luc
COBOL Software Modernization: From Principles to Implementation with the BLU AGE® Method

CHEN Ken
Performance Evaluation by Simulation and Analysis with Applications to Computer Networks

CLERC Maurice
Guided Randomness in Optimization
(Metaheuristics Set – Volume 1)

DURAND Nicolas, GIANAZZA David, GOTTELAND Jean-Baptiste, ALLIOT Jean-Marc
Metaheuristics for Air Traffic Management
(Metaheuristics Set – Volume 2)

MAGOULÈS Frédéric, ROUX François-Xavier, HOUZEAUX Guillaume
Parallel Scientific Computing

MUNEESAWANG Paisarn, YAMMEN Suchart
Visual Inspection Technology in the Hard Disk Drive Industry

2014

BOULANGER Jean-Louis
Formal Methods Applied to Industrial Complex Systems
Formal Methods Applied to Complex Systems: Implementation of the B Method

EXPOSITO Ernesto, DIOP Codé
Smart SOA Platforms in Cloud Computing Architectures

GARDI Frédéric, BENOIST Thierry, DARLAY Julien, ESTELLON Bertrand, MEGEL Romain
Mathematical Programming Solver based on Local Search

KRICHEN Saoussen, CHAOUACHI Jouhaina
Graph-related Optimization and Decision Support Systems

LARRIEU Nicolas, VARET Antoine
Rapid Prototyping of Software for Avionics Systems: Model-oriented Approaches for Complex Systems Certification

LAURAS Matthieu, ZELM Martin, ARCHIMÈDE Bernard, BÉNABEN Frédérick, DOUMEINGTS Guy
Enterprise Interoperability: Interoperability for Agility, Resilience and Plasticity of Collaborations

OUSSALAH Mourad Chabane
Software Architecture 1
Software Architecture 2

QUESNEL Flavien
Scheduling of Large-scale Virtualized Infrastructures: Toward Cooperative Management

RIGO Michel
Formal Languages, Automata and Numeration Systems 1: Introduction to Combinatorics on Words
Formal Languages, Automata and Numeration Systems 2: Applications to Recognizability and Decidability

SAINT-DIZIER Patrick
Musical Rhetoric: Foundations and Annotation Schemes

TOUATI Sid, DUPONT DE DINECHIN Benoit
Advanced Backend Code Optimization

2013

ANDRÉ Étienne, SOULAT Romain
The Inverse Method: Parametric Verification of Real-time Embedded Systems

BOULANGER Jean-Louis
Safety Management for Software-based Equipment

DELAHAYE Daniel, PUECHMOREL Stéphane
Modeling and Optimization of Air Traffic

FRANCOPOULO Gil
LMF — Lexical Markup Framework

GHEDIRA Khaled
Constraint Satisfaction Problems: CSP Formalisms and Techniques

GOVAERT Gérard, NADIF Mohamed
Co-Clustering: Models, Algorithms and Applications

LANDRAGIN Frédérick
Man–Machine Dialogue: Design and Challenges

LUCAS Laurent, LOSCOS Céline, REMION Yannick
3D Video: Models, From Capture to Diffusion

ROCHANGE Christine, UHRIG Sascha, SAINRAT Pascal
Time-Predictable Architectures

WAHBI Mohamed
Algorithms and Ordering Heuristics for Distributed Constraint Satisfaction Problems

ZELM Martin, VAN SINDEREN Marten, FERRAIRA PIRES Luis, DOUMEINGTS Guy
Enterprise Interoperability: Research and Applications in the Service-oriented Ecosystem

2012

ARBOLEDA Hugo, ROYER Jean-Claude
Model-Driven and Software Product Line Engineering

BLANCHET Gérard, DUPOUY Bertrand
Computer Architecture

BOULANGER Jean-Louis
Industrial Use of Formal Methods: Formal Verification
Formal Methods: Industrial Use from Model to the Code

CALVARY Gaëlle, DELOT Thierry, SÈDES Florence, TIGLI Jean-Yves
Computer Science and Ambient Intelligence

MAHOUT Vincent
Assembly Language Programming: ARM Cortex-M3 2.0: Organization, Innovation and Territory

MARLET Renaud
Program Specialization

SOTO Maria, SEVAUX Marc, ROSSI André, LAURENT Johann
Memory Allocation Problems in Embedded Systems: Optimization Methods

2011

BICHOT Charles-Edmond, SIARRY Patrick
Graph Partitioning

BOULANGER Jean-Louis
Static Analysis of Software: The Abstract Interpretation

CAFERRA Ricardo
Logic for Computer Science and Artificial Intelligence

KORDON Fabrice, HADDAD Serge, PAUTET Laurent, PETRUCCI Laure
Distributed Systems: Design and Algorithms
Models and Analysis in Distributed Systems

LORCA Xavier
Tree-based Graph Partitioning Constraint

RIDHA MAHJOUB A.
Progress in Combinatorial Optimization: ISCO2010

TRUCHET Charlotte, ASSAYAG Gerard
Constraint Programming in Music

VICAT-BLANC Pascale, GOGLIN Brice, GUILLIER Romaric,
SOUDAN Sébastien
Computing Networks: From Cluster to Cloud Computing

2010

AUBRUN Christophe, SIMON Daniel, SONG Ye-Qiong
Co-design Approaches for Dependable Networked Control Systems

AUDIBERT Pierre
Mathematics for Informatics and Computer Science

BABAU Jean-Philippe, BLAY-FORNARINO Mireille, CHAMPEAU Joël,
ROBERT Sylvain, SABETTA Antonino
Model Driven Engineering for Distributed Real-Time Systems: MARTE Modeling, Model Transformations and their Usages

BOULANGER Jean-Louis
Safety of Computer Architectures

SIGAUD Olivier, BUFFET Olivier
Markov Decision Processes in Artificial Intelligence

MONMARCHÉ Nicolas, GUINAND Frédérick, SIARRY Patrick
Artificial Ants

SOLNON Christine
Ant Colony Optimization and Constraint Programming

2009

FOURNIER Jean-Claude
Graph Theory and Applications: with exercises and problems

GUÉDON Jeanpierre
The Mojette Transform: theory and applications

JARD Claude, ROUX Olivier H.
Communicating Embedded Systems: Software and Design

LECOUTRE Christophe
Constraint Networks: Techniques and Algorithms

2008

BANÂTRE Michel, MARRON Pedro Jose, OLLERO Anibal, WOLITZ Adam
Cooperating Embedded Systems and Wireless Sensor Networks

MERZ Stephan, NAVET Nicolas
Modeling and Verification of Real-time Systems: Formalisms and Software Tools

PASCHOS Vangelis Th.
Combinatorial Optimization and Theoretical Computer Science: Interfaces and Perspectives

WALDNER Jean-Baptiste
Nanocomputers and Swarm Intelligence

2007

BENHAMOU Frédéric, JUSSIEN Narendra, O'SULLIVAN Barry
Trends in Constraint Programming

JUSSIEN Narendra
A to Z of Sudoku

2006

BABAU Jean-Philippe, CHAMPEAU Joël, GÉRARD Sébastien
From MDD Concepts to Experiments and Illustrations – DRES 2006

HABRIAS Henri, FRAPPIER Marc
Software Specification Methods: An Overview Using a Case Study

MURAT Cécile, PASCHOS Vangelis Th.
Probabilistic Combinatorial Optimization on Graphs

PANETTO Hervé, BOUDJLIDA Nacer
Interoperability for Enterprise Software and Applications: Proceedings of the Workshops and the Doctorial Symposium of the Second IFAC/IFIP I-ESA International Conference: EI2N, WSI, IS-TSPQ 2006

2005

GÉRARD Sébastien, BABAU Jean-Philippe, CHAMPEAU Joël
Model Driven Engineering for Distributed Real Time Embedded Systems

PANETTO Hervé
Interoperability of Enterprise Software and Applications: Workshops of the INTEROP-ESA 2005 International Conference (EI2N, WSI, ISIDI and IEHENA 2005)

Printed and bound by CPI Group (UK) Ltd, Croydon, CR0 4YY
16/09/2026
14963201-0001